Lotus Essences

An Encyclopaedia of Lotus Holistic Essences by
Julie Bowman
BFVEA Advanced Practitioner
BAFEP member
2nd Edition ©2022

Contents

Alphabetical List of All Essences.................. 238

Contents........................... 2
Dedication 5
This book 5
Copyright......................... 6
Acknowledgements............. 7
Introduction 9
Foreword to this edition by Clare G Harvey 11
Foreword to 1st Edition by Erik Pelham 12
The Use of Essences 14
    Essences 14
    Homeopathy.................15
    Herbal 15
    Aromatherapy 15
How to work with essences 17
    Dowsing.......................17
    Knowledge....................17
    Repertory.....................17
    Making an essence 18
    Taking essences 19
    Dosage 19
    Using this book 20
Journeying with Essences .. 21
Seaweed Essences............ 23
Flower Essences: 26

Apple Blossom 26
Bluebell..............................28
Buddleia.............................30
Camellia 31
Castor Oil Plant...................33
Cherry Blossom...................34
Christmas Cacti (Moon).......35
Christmas Cacti (Sun)..........37
Christmas Rose (cream).......39
Cornflower..........................41
Cranesbill 43
Creeping Buttercup 44
Elderflower 45
Forget me Not 47
Forsythia.............................49
Foxglove (pink) 51
Gingko-Biloba 52
Hazel Catkin 54
Hibiscus 55
Holly...................................56
Honesty 58
Inipi Moss 59
Japanese Azalea..................61
Japanese Azalea (Saki)........63
Kefalonia Bamboo 65
Kerria Japonica 66
Ladies Mantle 68
Lambs Ears........................69
Laurel................................70
Lotus 72
Mahonia 74
Mandrake 76
Medlar 78
Mimulus............................79
Money Plant 81
Montbretia 83
Nettle...............................85
New Zealand Flax 86
Orange Blossom 88
Ox Eye Daisy 91
Peace Lily 93
Pear 95

Peony 96
Pink Dog Rose 98
Pink/White Hawthorn 99
Plum 101
Pomegranate 102
Red Flowering Currant 104
Rhododendron 106
Rhubarb 108
Rosebay Willowherb 110
Rowan Berry 112
Rowan Blossom 113
Scabious 114
Self Heal 115
Snow Drop 117
Sycamore 119
Torbay Palm 121
Turkish-Filbert 123
Viburnum Burkwoodii 124
White Dog Rose 126
White Hawthorn 127
White Lilac 128
White Rambling Rose 131
White Sage 133
White Spirea 134
Wild Garlic 136
Willow 137
Wisteria 138
Yellow-Poppy 140

Essences made at the Field Ilkeston 141

Angelica seed 141
Belladonna 143
Black Cohosh 145
Black-Eyed-Susan (Rudbeckia) 147
Blackthorn 149
Boneset-Eupatorium-Perfoliatum 150
Borage 152
Calendula 154
Chamomile 156
Chicory 157
Clary-sage 159
Cowslip 160
Echinacea 161
Great-Burnet 163
Henbane 165
Iris-Germanic 167
Ivy 168
Lacy-Phacelia 170
Lavender 172
Marsh-Mallow 173
Mullein 174
Poke root 175
Pulsatilla 178
Rosemary 179
Scotch-Thistle 180
Scurvy-Grass 181
St-Johns-Wort 182
Tobacco 183
Valerian 184
Vipers-Bugloss 185
Yarrow 186

Fungus Essences 187
Turkey-Tail-Bracket-Fungus 187

Gem Essences 189
Basalt 189
Obsidian 191
Pearl 193

Channelled Essences 195
Bridging-the-Gap 195
Galactic-Configuration 197
Rainbow-Warrior 199

Seaweed Essences 201
Bifurcaria 201
Blackpool Mill 204
Caherdaniel Bladderwrack 206
Corallejo - Halimeda tuna . 207
Coralline 208
Derrynane Kelp 210

Iona 211
Kefalonia 213
Kelp 214
Kelp-holdfast 215
Mull 216
Oxwich Bay 218
Runswick-Bay.......................220
Sea Lettuce 221
Ulva 222
White-Bay 224
Seaweed Combination 226

Combination Essences..... 228

Back-On-Track 228
Chillax 229
Constellation Mix................230
Electro Protector 231
Exam Study 232
Helping Hands 233
Recuperation 235
Sunshine Lift 237

Alphabetical List of All Essences..........................238

Index of Keywords 241

Dedication

This book is dedicated to Dr Edward Bach, Clare G Harvey, Julian Barnard and Lila Devi.

Their inspiration, insights, dedication and love gave me hope and some of the tools I needed to enter into the magic.

This book

Julie Bowman BFVEA has been making essences since the mid 1990s and now has a varied collection of over 130 essences including combinations.
This book is and always will be a work in progress!
Feel free to comment and email suggestions/corrections to
julie@lotusholistic.com

Her husband, Rafe Nauen created the website as a database program, which the book was downloaded from. The editing was part of the final part of that process.

Copyright

Copyright © 2022 Julie Bowman

All rights reserved. No part of this publication may be reproduced, distributed, or transmitted in any form or by any means, including photocopying, recording, or other electronic or mechanical methods, without the prior written permission of the publisher, except in the case of brief quotations embodied in critical reviews and certain other non-commercial uses permitted by copyright law. For permission requests, write to the publisher, at the address below.

ISBN:

Hardback 979-8-4109-1165-8

Paperback 978-1-9849-5687-3

Front cover image by Julie Bowman.
Book design by Julie Bowman.
Database publishing & editing by Rafe Nauen.

Printed by KDP, Inc., in the United States of America and Europe

First edition 2018.
Updated Version 2020
This Edition 2022

Lotus Holistic

www.lotusholistic.com
Julie Bowman
+44 1332 280021
+44 7815 088180
julie@lotusholistic.com

Acknowledgements

Jan Stewart for her encouragement, love of essences and inspiration.

Jan Rose her many insights, interest in Essences and her in-depth work with 'Lotus Holistic.

My husband Rafe Nauen for his love, patience, encouragement and understanding, and for pulling together the database and publishing it all online and in this book for me.

To my many teachers who helped me with insights and understanding.

Clare G Harvey who has always encouraged me and for the extensive work we did together. It has taken me forward with my work with essences, and it has taught me that there are no limits to essences, just the limits we create.

BFVEA for their kindness and help along the way – they have always encouraged and supported me.

BAFAP who welcomed Lotus Holistic Essences into their fold.

To Weleda whose kind permission has enabled the Field essences to be birthed.

To all our Children and Grandchildren for their love support, encouragement and knowledge that essences help and support them.

To the spirits of the plants, gems, the land and the oceans without which, none of this would have been possible.

There are many more to whom I am grateful, who have supported and encouraged me and who have brought me to this point.

Introduction

Where and how did Lotus Holistic Essences evolve? Like many who come to use essences, my first encounter was with Rescue Remedy in 1984. Gradually I started to use other Bach essences and knew what a valuable tool they were. The effect was that they seemed to balance and calm my emotions.

Coming from a medical background I would think about the side effects of medicines. What I liked about essences that there were no side effects.

By the time I started to train as a reflexologist in 1993, I was well into using the essences, and started to dowse for clients. I was surprised that what came up was always relevant. Gradually this part of my life evolved. The second set I came across were the Spirit in Nature (formally Master Essences). I found these to be amazing - the simplicity really appealed to me, and they remain one of my favourite sets today.

Gradually the range of essences that I worked with expanded. They now include Bush, Baileys, Alaskan, Indigo, Petite Fleur, Light Bringer, Clare Harvey's range, and many others (not to mention Lotus Holistic!). I have been fortunate to have been taught by many pioneers and I also belong to the BFVEA which has always been very supportive.

In 2004 I was drawn to making an essence from 'Christmas Cacti'. At the time it was pure white, whereas now it is deep pink! It came up for clients again and again. I didn't realise the significance of this essence until much later. I made a second essence from the same plant later that year, but this time from the energy of the Moon. I didn't realise then, just how this range would grow!

A few years on when I had made other essences I realised that they needed a name. The origins of the name 'Lotus Holistic' were from my husband's former wife who sadly had passed away. She worked with essences herself, she had used the name Lotus Holistic. She bequeathed me her notes, her books, and her essences, so it seemed the right thing to do and call the essences Lotus Holistic Essences.

The magic that has filled my life is amazing. Essences are certainly full of magic and wonder. They reveal their secrets and always amaze me. Without essences I know that my journey would have been very different and much harder. At times they have saved my life.

Dr Bach left a legacy to which we owe a great gratitude.

Foreword to this edition by Clare G Harvey

It's been a pleasure to be witness to the joy and inspiration that Julie has drawn from Nature's "Flower & Plant World" and her subsequent development into a noteworthy essence producer not only of Flowers, and Gems but also her journey into essences from the sea.

Julie continually pushes the edges of exploration by developing and producing new essences. This book is an update to her original publication.

Flower Essences are now being recognized as an important healing modality. They are considered an essential "go-to" aid for their steadying effect when confronted by a confusing world of constant change.

Julie's Lotus Holistic Essences are a welcome contribution to the whole field of Vibrational Remedies.

Clare G Harvey

Harley Street Flower Essence Consultant, Formulator, and Author of the Practitioner's Encyclopaedia of Flower Remedies. Executive Director of the ISNS (International Science & Nutrition Society)

Foreword to 1st Edition by Erik Pelham

I am very excited to write this foreword for Julie's book as the Sea Weed Essences are a very important addition to the Wellbeing of the human race at this time. Also Julie's passion for finding natural solutions for all human and animal problems is awe inspiring ! The Essences themselves are powerful, yet subtle and perfect to help us with a whole range of relationship, health and general challenges that we face daily.

I will never forget the speed at which Julie's 'Oxwich Bay' sea essence healed some energy abuse I was suffering during a talk we both attended, and the way Julie intuitively pushed that essence towards me at exactly the right moment ! Why do the sea essences work so instantly and powerfully in relationship situations ? It is because they work straight into the 'interpersonal and group energy fields' that we share with others. By restoring the right resonance of our subtle bodies they eliminate intrusions of bad energy and any abuse or other bad effects we may be suffering because of these intrusions. In social and interpersonal relationship situations people have negative intrusions of energy from others all the time, but are generally unaware of it. The magic of Julie's sea essences is that they remedy this very quickly, restore wellbeing, discernment and harmony almost instantly and have no side effects or after effects, as some other modalities do.

With the help of these essences long term relationship problems can be healed and you can gain a wonderful new quality of life, and renewal of important relationships. I know this because I have been producing sea creature essences for

24 years now, which go out to around 30 countries around the world. Having entered the ocean worlds with the sea devas, dolphins and whales I have gained a strong and clear attunement with sea essences, and I always dreamed of someone making the wonderful sea plant essences. Then I met Julie at the BFVEA Gatherings and she instantly felt like a twin Soul on a Divine Mission to save humanity. My feelings at the first instant were correct and that is exactly what she has proved to be ! I personally love her essences and would recommend them to anyone in need of help both personally and in relationships with others, at an individual or group level.

Please read this book, get the essences and use them in your daily life – you will be amazed! Am I biased – of course I am ! The power of the sea essences to improve our daily lives is undisputable and the relevance of Julie's essences to our everyday problems is very clear. We just need to take that leap of faith and will to embrace the most primal power to heal in our world, that of the life energies coming through the oceans and seas – the power of Lotus Holistic Essences.

Thanks be to OM.

Love,

Erik

Erik Pelham

The Use of Essences

Many people get confused with the differences between essences, homeopathy, herbal medicines, and aromatherapy.

I decided to include an explanation about each to bring some clarity.

Essences

Essences literally are the energetic imprint of the plant, flower, gem, spirit of the land taken into water.

They are safe, non-addictive can be used with any other medication and any medical condition, and can e safely used on children, babies, animals, with plants and on land.

"Flower essences are tools for transformation, catalysts for change.

They work by enhancing the positive aspects of the qualities of mind emotion and personality. By flooding a person with positive qualities, the negative aspects or lack of positive are dissolved, and health is restored." Source Dr Tressider's website

Through ingesting some of the plants' energetic essences, we give our bodies a model of new integration we can then use to build new patterns, helping ourselves to heal – on emotional, psychological and spiritual, as well as physical levels. These gentle modes of healing are clearly the way of the future. Source Buffalo Woman Comes Singing by Brook Medicine Eagle

Homeopathy

"Homeopathy is a natural form of medicine used by over 200 million people worldwide to treat both acute and chronic conditions. It is based on the principle of 'like cures like'. In other words, a substance taken in small amounts will cure the same symptoms it causes if taken in large amounts" Source: British Homeopathic Association website

Herbal

"Medical Herbalists make use of plants whose traditional uses are backed up by modern scientific research and clinical trials. A Qualified Medical Herbalist has a BSc or equivalent in Herbal Medicine, has studied orthodox medicine as well as plant medicine and is trained in the same diagnostic skills as a GP. However, Herbalists take an holistic approach to illness, treating the underlying cause of disease rather than just the symptoms. They are able to prescribe herbal remedies to be used alongside other medication and treatments, and many patients are referred to a Herbalist by their GP for treatment."

Herbal Medicine is suitable for people of any age, including children, who respond especially well to the gentle actions of herbs. Each patient is treated as an individual – a Medical Herbalist recognises that no two patients are the same. Source: The National Institute of Medical Herbalists

Aromatherapy

"Aromatherapy, also referred to as Essential Oil therapy, can be defined as the art and science of utilizing naturally extracted

aromatic essences from plants to balance, harmonize and promote the health of body, mind and spirit." Source: National Association for Holistic Aromatherapy

How to work with essences

Working with essences - there is a whole process that takes place.

Dowsing

When I first started working with essences, I had no knowledge base at all so I used a pendulum to find what was needed. Then I would read what I had picked. To my amazement I invariably found that the results were appropriate.

Knowledge

As time went by, I decided it would be good to gain a knowledge base, so attended courses and did a practitioner's course. I found the whole process totally fascinating and I still do.

Repertory

Of course, there is always repertories (this book is one) which is a good way of finding an essence that fits.

These days there are also various methods of working with the intuition. As I have already mentioned there is the dowsing method.

Photos are another way some essence producers use. They have had photos of their essences made into cards. You can pick a card and often the card picked will be relevant.

We can also scan the essences and often there is an energetic pull and again totally appropriate.

Of course, there are many other ways of which you may discover for yourself.

Making an essence

When I make an essence for a client. I may have some information about what the client is encountering. So, I may work from an intuitive perspective, bringing in the knowledge and using the repertory.

I often work blind so that just intuition and dowsing give me the results. I may also ask before I dowse for an essence to support with specific issues. It always delights and surprises how relevant the essences that come up are.

Sometimes, I end up with 20 essences or more, this may stay in a single dosage bottle, or it may divide up into more than one bottle. I will dowse to see what essences go into which bottle and this can work in various ways. I see this a bit like an orchestra with different elements coming together in the mix. Sometimes one essence will give the person what they need, at other times there may be many essences that are working together in harmony. Some may be supporting in the background. The magic just goes on and on.

Taking essences

Essences can be administered in many ways.

They can be taken orally - 5 drops onto the tongue 3x daily. If a person has issues with alcohol I will use apple vinegar, salt, glycerine, red shiso or just water. With just water it won't keep as long so it is best kept in the fridge for up to 4 weeks.

Straight into water hot or cold, drinking throughout the day.

They can be made it up into a spray. I would use vodka and water mixed. 40% vodka 60% spring water. Aromatherapy oils can be added; however, you need to be a qualified aromatherapist to administer this mix.

You can rub them onto the skin a few drops on the wrists, tummy or temples.

Essences can be added to creams and again a few drops mixed into the cream and rub onto the skin.

Another really nice way of working with them is to put them into the bath 7 drops giving it a good swoosh round.

Dosage

The number of drops which go into an essence will vary with different ranges.

With Lotus holistic 5 drops is the recommended dosage 3 times a day. Clients will at time administer them more with no ill effects. Three times is the minimum dosage that has the most beneficial results.

As average the dosage bottle should last for a month. Clients working with essences on a regular basis find this a really effective support mechanism for themselves.

Using this book

Using this book alongside the 'Lotus Holistic' essences give you a really clear picture of what the essences are for.

Included at the back of the book is an index which can be referenced by keywords.

i.e. Focus will reference Christmas Cacti sun and the page number

The book can also be enjoyed giving you an insight into how magical and amazing their world is. Good luck on your journey.

Journeying with Essences

Back in 1984 after the birth of my first daughter, like many new mum's I felt out of my depth.

A friend gave me a little bottle of Rescue remedy, I found the magic of this remedy so effective it became part of my life and like with homeopathy, I was hooked. I liked the fact that they were safe and worked really well. I started to look at the other Bach Essences and gradually owned all 38. Using the dowsing method found I could mix remedy's and found their effect on the emotions to be highly effective.

I trained as a nurse and was, of course, using conventional medicines, I was delighted to find something that resonated so deeply and beautifully.

In 1993 as I trained as a Reflexologist and started to use essences on clients using dowsing. I found that they really helped clients. Around this time, I was introduced to the 'Spirit in Nature' (Masters' Essences). Still one of my favourite sets, they are very simple with only 20 essences in the set. They have a beautiful feminine quality to them.

Essences help us get to know who we are and to travel deep within to our core. They help us to grow in wisdom. They give us a sense of peace which is something at the heart of who we are. However, life brings with it challenges and pushes us through having to find resources within ourselves. At these points essences can benefit us by showing what issues we are working with. They can help to bring clarity, strength and get us back on track. There have been many times over the past 30 years when they have literally saved me, giving me hope and bringing me back to centre.

There will always be challenges and as spiritual beings having a human experience part of that journey is to experience emotional challenges. Over the years my path has taken me to places that has been harrowing and from these experiences I have grown and developed.

What my journey has given me are tools, and essences are a major part of those tools. Meditation is also part of my spiritual practice as well as sweat lodges, using the Medicine Wheel. The use of essences has certainly made me more comfortable with who I am, offering a support and insight, helping me to listen to my own inner voice. They help us to get to the heart of the matter, teaching us to be kind to ourselves. When I hear about being self-centred there are two ways to look at this. Being in the centre of ourselves is one way. We can value ourselves, which entails self-care, respect for ourselves, loving ourselves and this all increases our self-worth. If we deny this, then our journeys are doomed. Learning to value myself has been a big part of my journey. Essences have certainly helped me work through the layers and continue to do so.

Essences have an energetic imprint of something which is exquisitely beautiful. They hold a blueprint and they hold light. They take the imprint of the flower, gem, seaweed, or whatever the essences energy holds. The magic become part of who we are, bringing to us aspects of who we are.

In 2004 I was drawn to one of my house plants Christmas Cacti and made an essence by the sun method. Later calling it Christmas Cacti Sun. it is one of the most important essences that I have ever made. Later that year I also made an essence from the moon - Christmas Cacti Moon.

It wasn't until 2009 that more essences started to follow. Rhododendron in May of that year which is all about boundaries. I had remarried and was living with six teenagers, so boundaries became extremely important! The next came soon after - New Zealand Flax for heart to heart communication which looking back I can see why!

In the early days I made essences from house plants and out of my garden but as time has gone by, I have gone further afield. Since 2013 I have been making essences from a variety of seaweeds.

I am also very fortunate to have Jan Rose - a really good friend and colleague (who I was introduced to by Jan Stewart.)

Seaweed Essences

In 2011 the essences took a surprising turn. A friend asked me about making seaweed essences! I looked at her surprised and really dismissed the whole idea. In 2013 two years later Angela turned up with six seaweeds. So, I dried them out and took them home.

Later that year I was going on retreat to Mull and was pushed to take the seaweeds with me. I was quite irritated by this. It was a retreat I was going on!! in the end I concluded that I just needed to get on with it.

Taking the seaweeds with me was an interesting experience. Looking back, I went through some emotionally harrowing experiences. However, it expanded me as I went through a range of emotions - some of which were really hard.

I never know what an essence is about until after the event. When I read my notes about the original six seaweed essences it isn't surprising what I encountered. I made the essences over the course of three days. On the second day I saw the most amazing rainbow. The weather over the three days was extremely changeable.

I realised that although the seaweed essences would work on an individual basis, they wanted to work as a combination too. It was during this period that I was meditating one evening and Neptune appeared! He was so angry about how we were treating the planet. I apologised and vowed to do some work. By March 2014 I had made a combination Seaweed Essence (with the addition of Pearl essence) which I started to give away for people to work with in ceremony and ritual to honour the earth and the water.

Since the original six seaweed essences I have gone on to make more seaweed essences and these too have become part of the combination. The work they are doing is just delightful.

I have given well over a thousand bottles away for which I never charge, as I feel they are playing a really important role. The seaweed essences stand alone as amazing individual essences. However, as a combination they are proving to be very powerful. They have been used with the Warriors Call earth healing work. People have taken them all over the world, doing ceremony and rituals.

I get lots of feedback and am astonished that I am part of all this!

Lotus Holistic continues to grow and evolve and is proving to be an amazing journey.

Looking back over the past 30 years and seeing how all the essences are developing is truly amazing. To know that I am part of that process as a kind of midwife, is extraordinary.

Flower Essences:

Apple Blossom

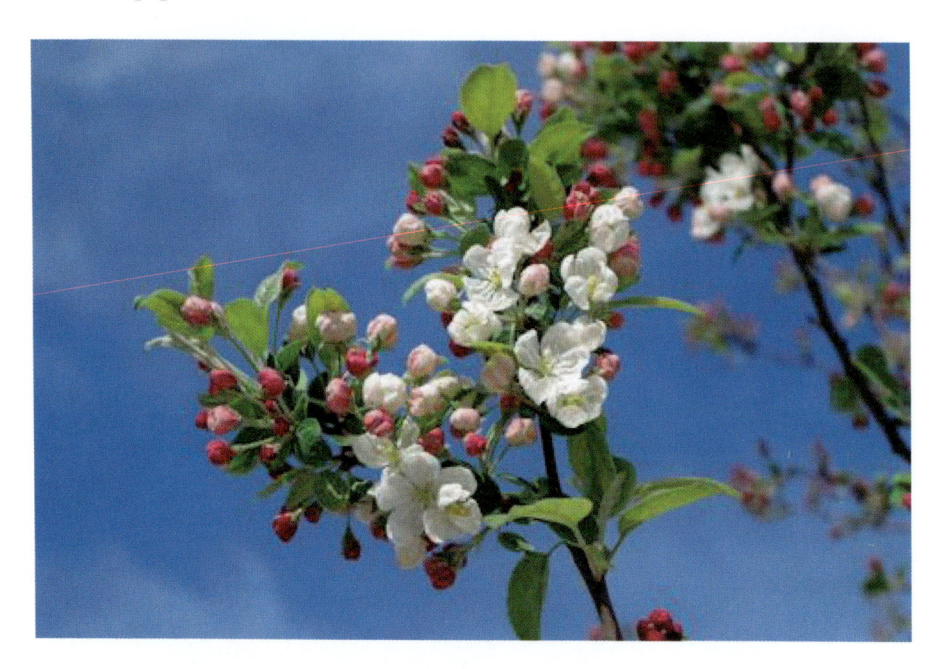

Keywords: birth, joy, renewal, patience, tenacity, motivator, strength, wisdom, growth, focus, habit breakers, ancestral, addictions, habits

Indications: Renewal, bringing with it growth.
Its really good to support the breaking of habits.
For building in new practices and good habits e.g. gym, meditation

This essence brings with it renewal. Qualities of self-love. It's like being born anew which brings with it a sense of Joy.

Healing Qualities: *Jan Roses insights*
Good when learning something new and needing to practice over and over again e.g. athletes musicians, dancers, 'Practice makes

perfect'.
Helps with sticking with something you might find difficult and initially unrewarding. Keeping going even if you can't yet see tangible results. It gives tenacity and strength to see things through to the end.
Delayed gratification. Not losing heart and keeping motivation going and the final goal in sight.

Tapping into ancestral strength and help, going back to your roots to find ways to keep moving forward.
Looking at patterns and cycles in your own linage e.g. when in their lives your ancestors at their most powerful and successful? At what stages in their lives did a significant event occur? When familiar patterns and seeing how positivity can be applied.

Notes: Budding blossoming fruiting dropping dormancy and repeat over and over.
This essence was made from a really old apple tree that had loads of dead wood cut from it very little of the tree was left. Yet in spite of this it put flowers out. I came back from being away and the flowers had finished. Yet a couple of weeks later it gave more flowers. It was from these late flowers that I made the essence. Jan's insights certainly made sense. *Jan Rose's essence*
Solid in the hand.
Planted grounded.
Roots pushing their way firmly and determinedly down and across, anchoring into the earth.

once properly anchored, the life force forges a path.

Bluebell

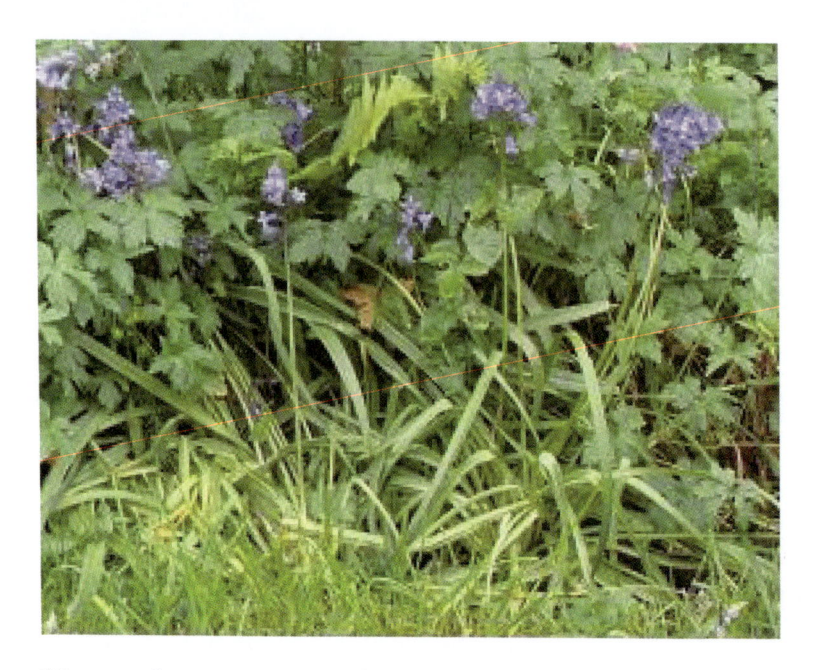

Keywords: acceptance, change, safe, heart, go with the flow, fear, flustered, authentic, on course, purpose,

Indications: Crown chakra, ,3rd eye chakra, heart chakra, root Chakra.
For the heart chakra, works on fear, enables you to accept change, go with the flow, for feeling safe. Enjoy the day enjoy the moment.

Healing Qualities: This essence is about living authentically from the heart. Dispensing with masks and pretences. Feeling secure enough to be yourself and live as dictated by your Divine plan, not as dictated by your fellow man.

For following your heart, feeding your soul.

It is good to use when people are thrown by continual and or dramatic changes. It helps them to feel safe and secure even in the midst of what appears chaotic and gives them the ability to see it as an opportunity rather than a threat. Accepting change, understanding that life does change going with the flow of life not resisting it.

Notes: *Jan Rose's Insights*
used this when I felt flustered and aggrieved over an employer and underpaying me, couldn't settle to anything and finding it difficult to settle at night. Took this for 24 hours and found it brilliant. Stopped feeling wobbly and upset, felt calmer. I also realised that to resolve this problem would need to remember to 'stay in the heart 'it would be easier to let emotions cloud my judgement and lead me to let fly at the people involved which would no doubt cause a huge rift. Helped me to understand that it is probably crossed wires, not some evil intent to rip me off!! Clairaudience

Buddleia

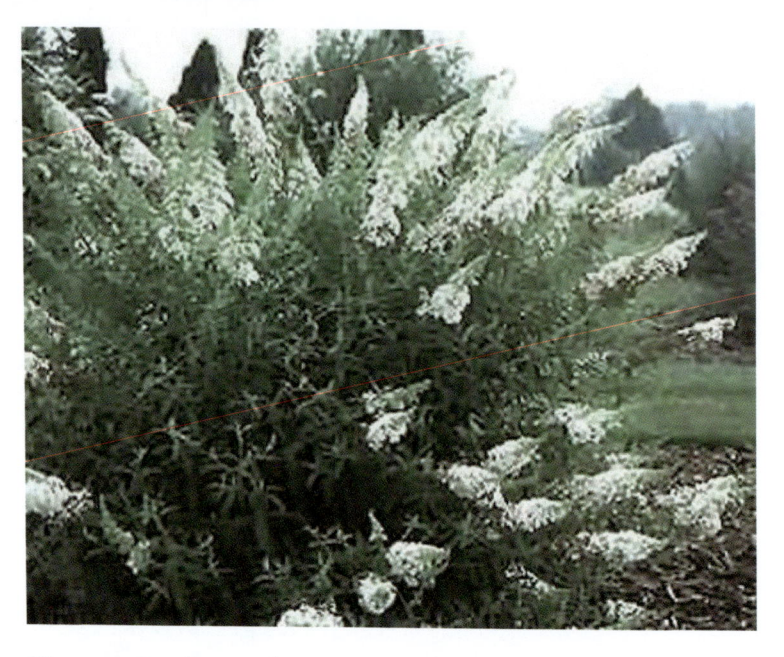

Keywords: depression, ancestral, confidence, pattern breaker, nurtures, lifts, feed the spirit, addictions, resilience

Indications: This essence is about confidence.
It's about letting go of old Ancestral patterns of destruction.
It helps with nurturing ourselves.
where life has challenged you leaving you feeling raw and totally out of sorts and raw.

Healing Qualities: As an essence it will bring deep nurturance, lifting the spirit
Aiding us to fight back face challenges, helping to become confident in life again

Notes: Buddleia will die back, or take a herd cut back and regrow. There is a resilience's to buddleia in its gesture.

Camellia

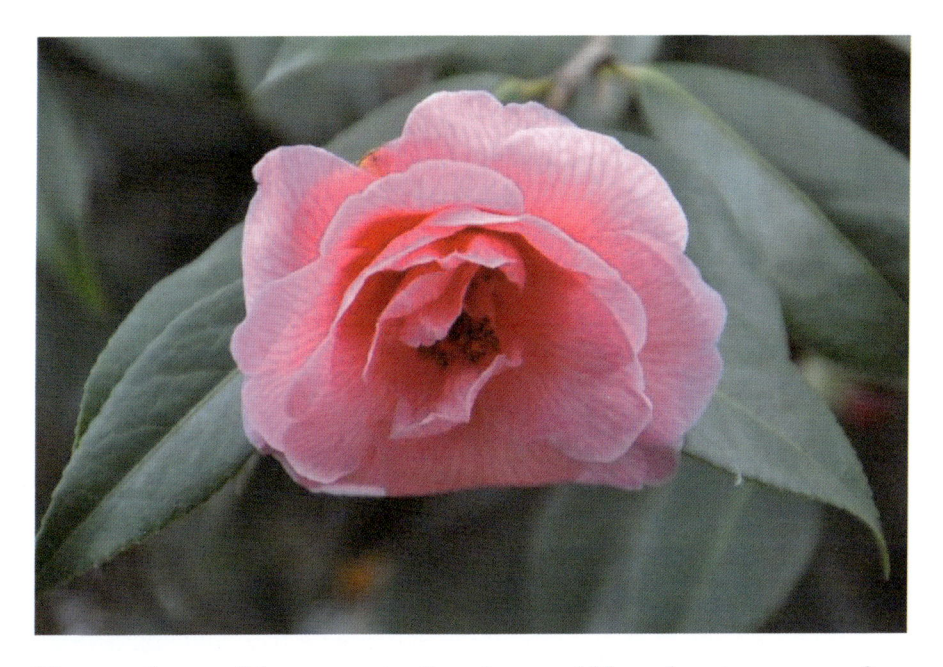

Keywords: confidence, protection, love, self-love heart, peace, safe, trust, stuck, soul, spirit,
heart-break,

Indications: Eyes, Ears, Temples Brow chakra.
Helps get to the 'Heart of the Matter'
This essence feels like it coats your Aura , protective.
Helps us to feel safe in our journey.
It gives us the spirit of adventure. Trusting in the journey.

Healing Qualities: This essence is useful for when you are exploring unfamiliar territory, whether that is physical, emotional or spiritual. It helps you to trust that you will have a safe passage. Spirit of adventure and enterprise. Nothing ventured, nothing gained. Understanding that it is not the destination that is important, it is the actual journey and experience.
When stuck, it helps you to take that first all-important small step, trust the process and allow it all to unfold.

Notes: *Jan Rose's insights*
Looking through a telescope at sea, harbour, seagulls and a red and white lighthouse. Sunny and tranquil, then gradually it becomes greyer with a choppy sea. Gulls set up wheeling and screeching. There is a storm blowing up. The tide moving out reveals a rough shingle beach. I notice a large brown shelled crab moving sideways up the shingle. It heads away from the sea, up the beach and up some steps. It continues across the pavement and then the road. It takes itself off into some sand dunes.
There it stays, fully enjoying the experience of its new environment. It just sits waiting through the night in the rain.
In the morning, the brown crab makes its way back across the road and pavement, down the steps and back onto the beach. There it waits for the morning tide, until the waves reach out and take it back out to sea.

Castor Oil Plant

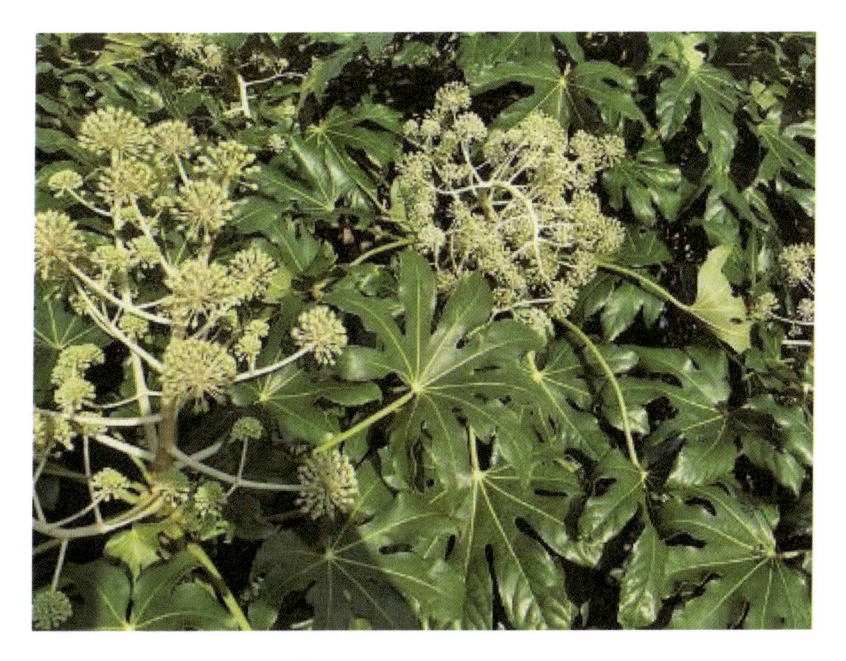

Keywords: focus, light, congested energy, regenerates

Indications: This essence draws stuff together.
Breaks up any congested energy. Stimulating and regenerating the energy field in a gentle and effective way. This essence harnesses the energy of light because of this process.

Healing Qualities: Castor Oil has some amazing healing qualities. Edgar Cayce spoke highly of Castor Oil. Castor Oil Plant' colloquial name is Palma Christi (Palm of Christ)

Cherry Blossom

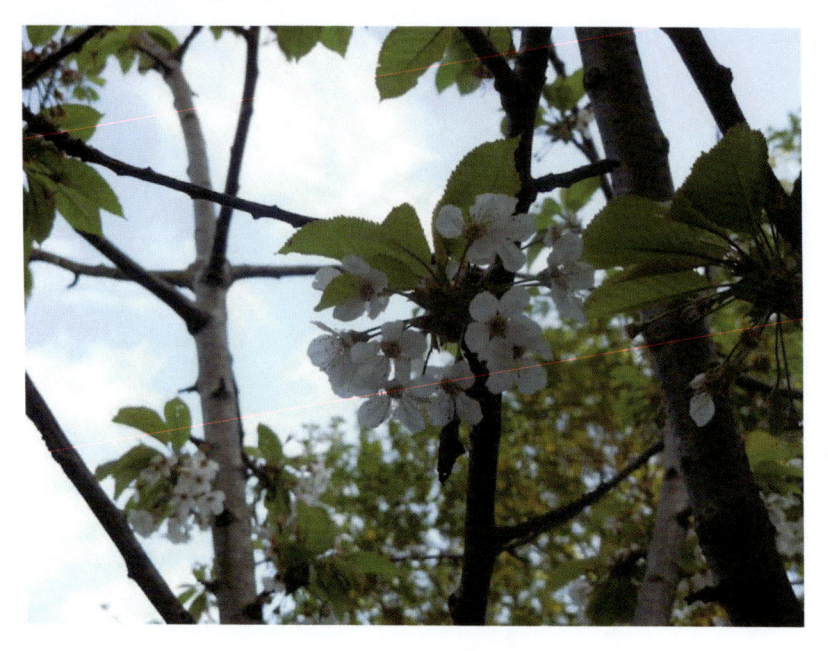

Keywords: angelic, happiness, lightness, joy, good will, upbeat, uplifts, grumpy, gloomy, dismal, irritable,

Indications: out of sorts, bear with a sore head, dark cloud, engenders good will,

Healing Qualities: "Ding-dong-merrily-on-high" is the song that came into my head the first time I connected with this essence. It has an angelic feel to it no surprises. Cherry essence brings joy and a sense of lightness. Leaving you feeling upbeat and uplifted.

Christmas Cacti (Moon)

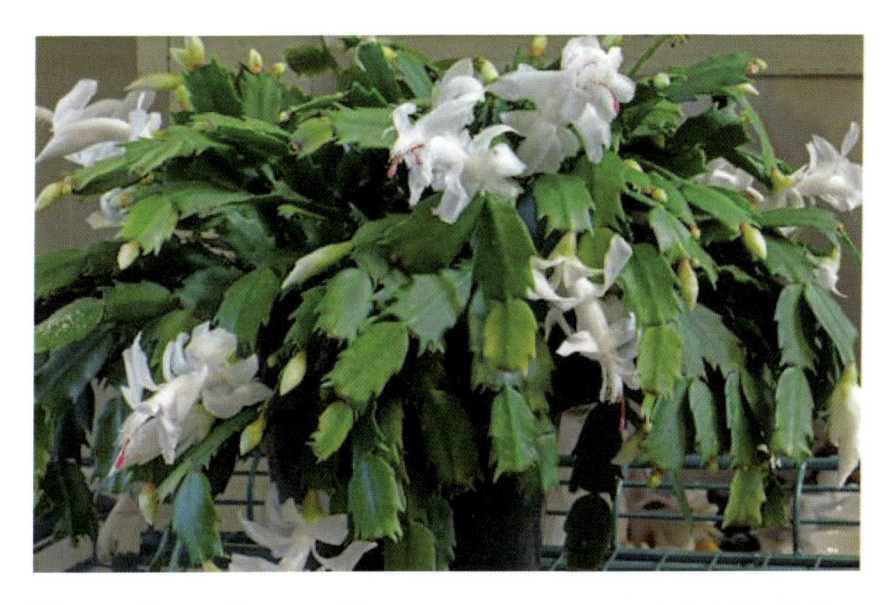

Keywords: settles, serenity, peace, courage, constraint, limitations, connects, settling at night, meditation, restrictions

Indications: Heart chakra,
Helps us to break free of constraints and limitations, which are imposed on us. This essence helps us feel connected.
Good for meditation, It gives a sense of peace. This is a remedy that settles and helps with difficulty settling at night.

Healing Qualities: Breaking free of constraints and limitations, particularly those imposed by others (be it by individuals, organisations or governments) and inspiring others to do the same. Leading by example. Unity. Strength in numbers. Finding kindred spirits. Solidarity.
The courage to go your own away and the trust that there are others out there like you and that you will all find each other in time.
I know some clients find this helpful with difficulty settling at night helping to be more rested.

Notes: *Jan Rose's insights*

Full moon over a dark sea. Rigged sailing ship moves across the water in front of the low moon. Anchors close to the base of cliffs. Rowing boat leaves it and moves across towards the land. Boat bumping as they come ashore, flashlights partially illuminate the scene. Voices. The men move inland.

Large dark creature bound and tied heavily with ropes. Men shouting and pulling and pushing and trying to force it down to the beach. Distressed, afraid, bellowing and resisting. Can hear answering calls from another creature further inland. The men continue to pull, hit and goad the distraught creature towards the sea. The men jump into their boat and row back towards their ship, dragging the reluctant creature behind. It is long necked, rather like archetypal images of the Loch Ness monster. On land, the men were the masters. In water, the creature is the master of its own element. Despite its restraints, it becomes swift, agile and graceful. It dives silently below the waves, dragging its tormentors and their boat with it. Surfaces and dives again. The boat bobs up empty, oars adrift and men scattered and floundering in the sea. The ropes that had been used to bind the creature float uselessly in the dark water.

The creature dives and surfaces effortlessly, shaking off the energetic effects of its imprisonment. Pays no attention to the men thrashing around impotently in the sea. Calls joyfully to the other creature incarcerated on the land; its voice strong and deep. The other creature replies. Back and forth they call to each other, encouraging and gaining strength and confidence with each round. From the land comes the sound of crashing and splintering wood, with the calls becoming louder and still stronger. The second creature emerges from the darkness of the land, lumbering clumsily but quickly down to the sea. Enters the ocean with a resounding splash.

The creatures greet each other in delight. Swim swiftly and gracefully away together, perfectly synchronised, towards the rising (now orange) moon. Calling together in joyous unison, gaining in strength as they go. Faintly, from other directions, more calls can be heard (albeit faintly). The creatures are linking up and communicating from around the globe, encouraging each other.

Christmas Cacti (Sun)

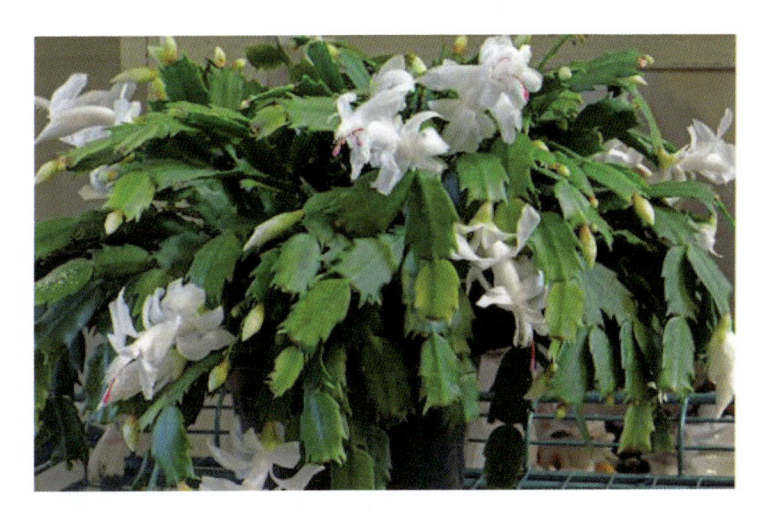

Keywords: anchor, energy, manifests, realigns, connection, focus, grounding, harmonisation, Helping Hands

Indications: Processing and assimilation. Base chakra, isn't functioning as it should.

it realigns the chakras
This remedy is excellent for focus. Excellent when you float off, really good for grounding.

When you have had your circuits blown and need to ground and realign. A really good remedy for when life has severely impacted.

Healing Qualities: Christmas Cacti sun is included in Helping Hands. Excellent for those who float off, never putting any proper roots down, often unable to manifest what they need or to make things happen in their lives.
It is an excellent essence to anchor, manifest, claim our place in the world. Meeting your own needs, rather than expecting others to do it for you.
Really good when there has been unpleasant events which has blown your circuits, and you need realigning. It brings the physical, emotional, mental, and spiritual back into alignment.

For those who are ambivalent or undecided about remaining on the planet, it will help you to take your place. It is a great energiser. This essence is for those who want to access and use higher energies, but without doing the groundwork. It helps to give us understanding that spirituality comes from the feet up. Useful for those who have had their circuits blown.

It is good to ground if a person is prone to float, who find it hard to put down roots. This will help to manifest what they need to make things happen in their lives and help connect to the Heavens. For those who are ambivalent about being here and remaining on this planet.

It helps to anchor, manifest, claim your place in the world. Meeting your own needs, rather than expecting others to do it for you.
It is a healer in its own right. Physically, mentally, emotionally, and spiritually. It reconnects and brings everything back into line. It is a great harmoniser.

Notes: 3rd eye. Feet. Roots growing from the soles of the feet into the ground. Coming up through the plant and burst out of the flower into the waiting blue sky and bright sun. Base chakra where this is not functioning as it should. The flowers on the Christmas Cacti at the time of making this essence were white. Gradually over time they have turned pink and are now a beautiful dark facia red.

Christmas Rose (cream)

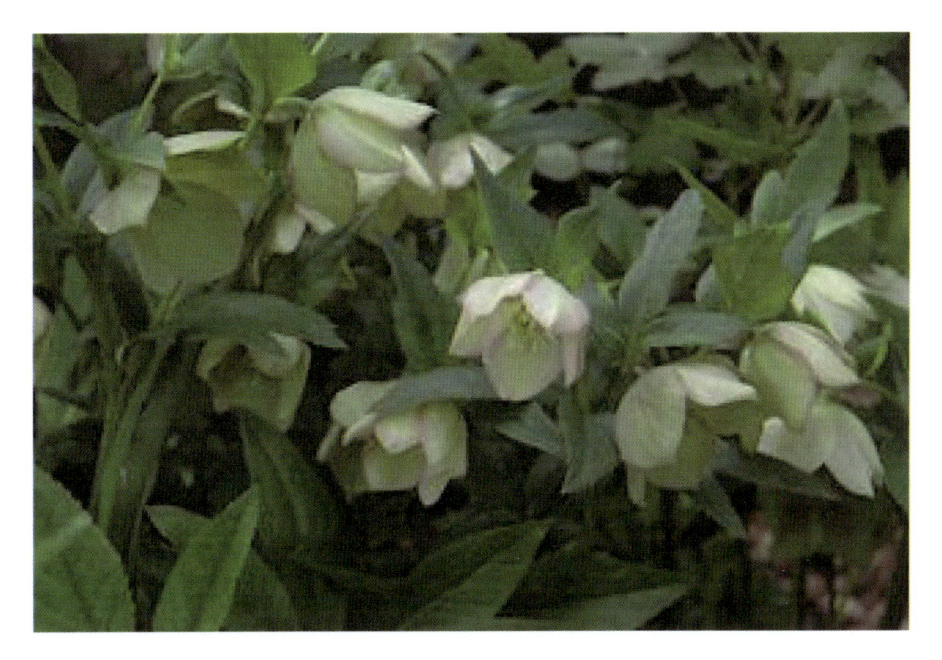

Keywords: holding, settles, sooths, connection, peace, abundance, optimism, gratitude, joy, reflect, pregnancy support, patience

Indications: lively glad to be alive, 'joie de vivre' Effervescence. Indicated when head too full.

Brings a sense of an abundance joy.

Healing Qualities: it is a good supportive essence for pregnancy. When we look at the gesture of this beautiful flowers they have a humility about them, a grace. They have a spiritual connection.
I made this essence when I was due to speak at the Flower essence conference. It simply held me. Its beautiful energy held me I felt calm and clear, during the build-up and during the talk. I gave it to a college of mine and she said the same.

Especially good if someone has had an unsuccessful pregnancy after previous difficulty but is tense and apprehensive, unable to truly believe that all will be well and come to fruition. Supports the process to relax and enjoy any future developments happily and securely in the moment. (For this purpose, it would combine well with pomegranate)

It helps you reflect on your journey, seeing how far you have come.

Notes: *Jan Rose Insights 10/09/17 Lively and glad to be alive! Optimism. Joie de vivre. Effervescence.*
There has been a hard time germinating an idea a creation, the difficult slow push through solid ground, but at long last it has emerged into warming light of day. Good for when you realise just how far you have come on your journey and how well you have actually done.
Especially good if someone has become pregnant after previous difficulty but is tense and apprehensive, unable to truly believe that all will be well and come to fruition. Enables her to relax and enjoy the pregnancy and live happily and securely in the moment. (For this purpose, would combine well with pomegranate)

Cornflower

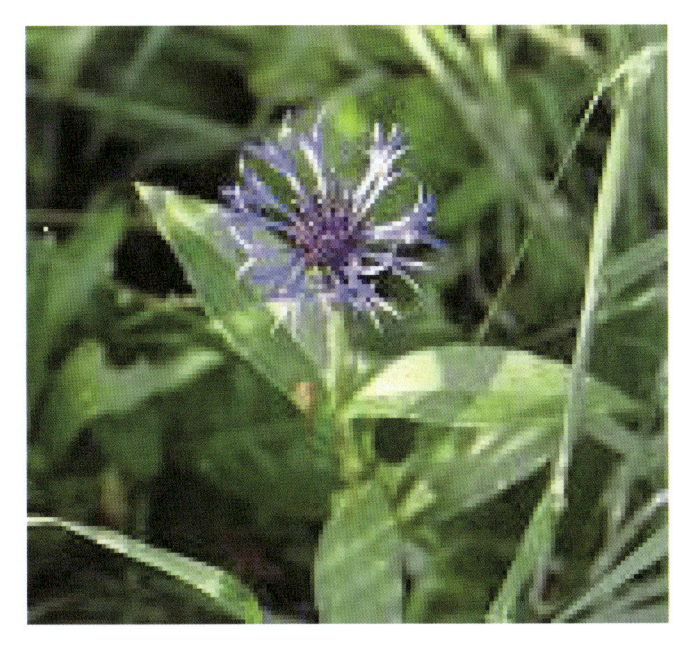

Keywords: focus, awareness, kindness, humility, aspirations, aims, obsessive, workaholics,

Indications: crown throat, throat chakra,
Enhances clear sight. Empowering and gives focus.
It can be used as a cleanser for scrying tools. Speaking one's truth useful for stressed workaholics and people who are very single minded.

Healing Qualities: This is an essence that focuses on many levels, helping us to see clearer and speak our truth with conviction and clarity.
Jan Roses insights
Being able to enjoy the fun and laughter of social interactions and situations but getting distracted or side-tracked by them; always keeping in mind your own aims and aspirations.

Being in the world but not of it

Enjoying the physical and the material aspects of this world but not being seduced or overtaken by them.
Despite our physicality remaining aware that we are part of something much bigger and eternal. We are more than we see here.

Spiritual awareness and openness to guidance Always aiming as high as we can, but with integrity, kindness, respect humility and awareness. It is possible to succeed but still remain a genuine and spirit led being. These types can obsess about work, good for business people.

Notes: *Jan Roses insights*
Strong steady deep pulsating energy.
Growing upwards.
Blue flower swaying gently in the breeze, in a field on the sunny summers day. Looking upwards and striving towards the sun.
very vibrant colours

Vervain/ Black eyed Susan types.

Cranesbill

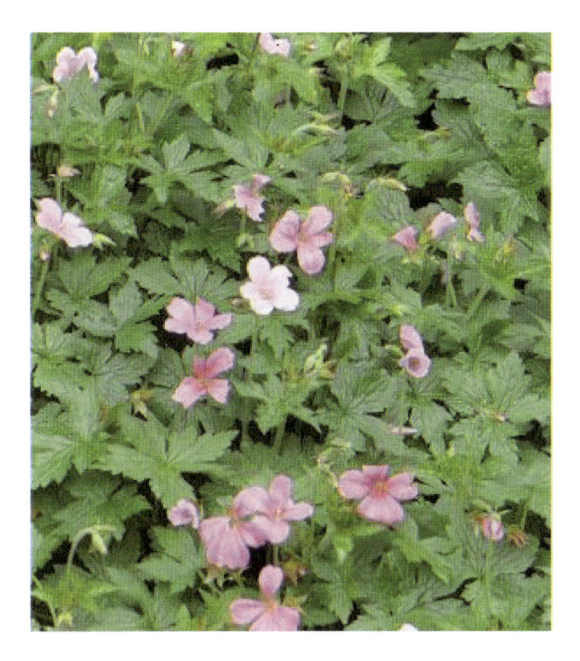

Keywords: centring, protection, aura, support, soul, strength, assertive, confidence, heart chakra,

Indications: Good when working with people. Keeps the energy intact preventing any leaking or being drained, protecting the Aura and personal energies.
Assertive when needed. It also has a gentle strength about it energy.

Healing Qualities: Helps to see the bigger picture. It sooths a troubled soul.
It is a good essence to take before treating clients as it will protect your energetic space. Take before talking to or working with clients. Helping us to be assertive when needed
For staying in the heart chakra whilst dealing with others but maintaining the ability to preserve yourself the gentle strength that this essence has certainly helps with this .

Creeping Buttercup

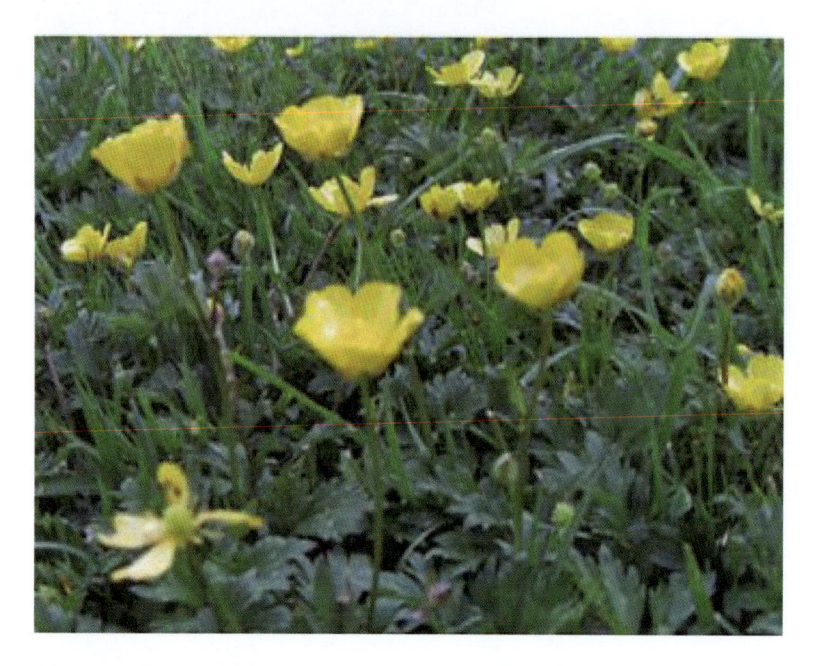

Keywords: self-love, nurturing, uplifts, deep sadness, depression, melancholia,

Indications: It brings happiness to the heart chakra. Creeping buttercup is about love learning to love the self.

Healing Qualities: It creates a chain reaction of good stuff. Helps us to feel comfortable with ourselves.
This lovely essence uplifts. Creeping buttercup is about love learning to love the self. It brings happiness to the heart chakra, and good stuff.
Helps you to learn to love the self. By loving ourselves more easily it helps to love others, being kind to ourselves and loving ourselves is where it all starts. It uplifts, bringing feelings of happiness connecting and brings about a chain reaction
The heart shaped leaves indicate the heart chakra.

Elderflower

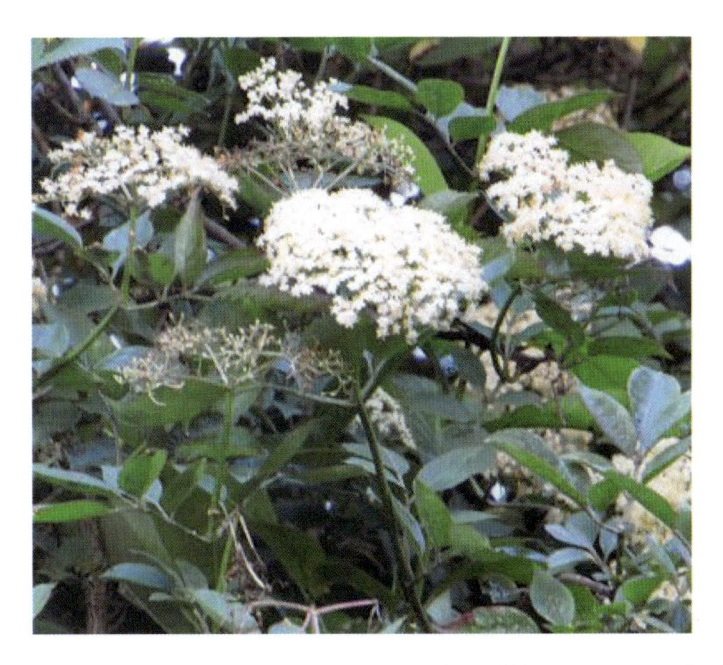

Keywords: acceptance, ancestral, resilience, strength, flexibility, adapt, procrastinate, fear, turmoil, commotion

Indications: Elderflower is for Working with how it is!! Putting you into a 'can do frame of mind.
This essence seems to have a lot to do with 'Resilience' and weathering the storms of life.
Good for procrastination or afraid to tackle a task that will bring upheaval.

Healing Qualities: Elderflower is a strong essence, helping in situations that challenge us and worrying about challenges that life brings. If this is the case, Elderflower will help us find a different way to deal with situations.
Good for when you are procrastinating or afraid to tackle a task that will bring upheaval.
It is helpful when in the midst of inevitable or necessary turmoil.

This essence has a lot of strength in it. It is indicated as an Ancestral healer.

Notes:
Strong almost painful feel in left hand. Firm hold. Heart. Flat land gridded with canals. Symmetry and man made order in the middle of nature. Lots of activity within this enclave, much busyness. High fence rings this vast watery metropolis. Bare land from the fence to the base of the mountains. Long horned mountain goat watches from the base of a mountain. Bounds across the no-mans-land and leaps the high fence bordering the settlement. Explores with interest, trotting around looking at everything.

People back away, terrified of this inquisitive intruder. Arm themselves with big sticks and oars and run down the straight lines of the canals to try to attack him. The goat dodges nimbly this way and that, bounding over waterways and across any obstacles, completely perplexing his pursuers.

He always remains alert and one jump ahead of the mob, but still manages to see what he wants to see and explore their territory. He is aware of their intentions but not in fear of them. He examines and explores with interest without allowing the fearful and aggressive hordes to disrupt or interfere with him.

When he has seen all that he came to see, he nonchalantly hops onto the roof of a boat and uses it as a springboard back over the fence. Once over, he turns to face the still overexcited noisy crowd on the other side. Even after he has calmly moved out of their view, the people are still jittery and nervous, peering through the fence in dread in case he has returned.

Forget me Not

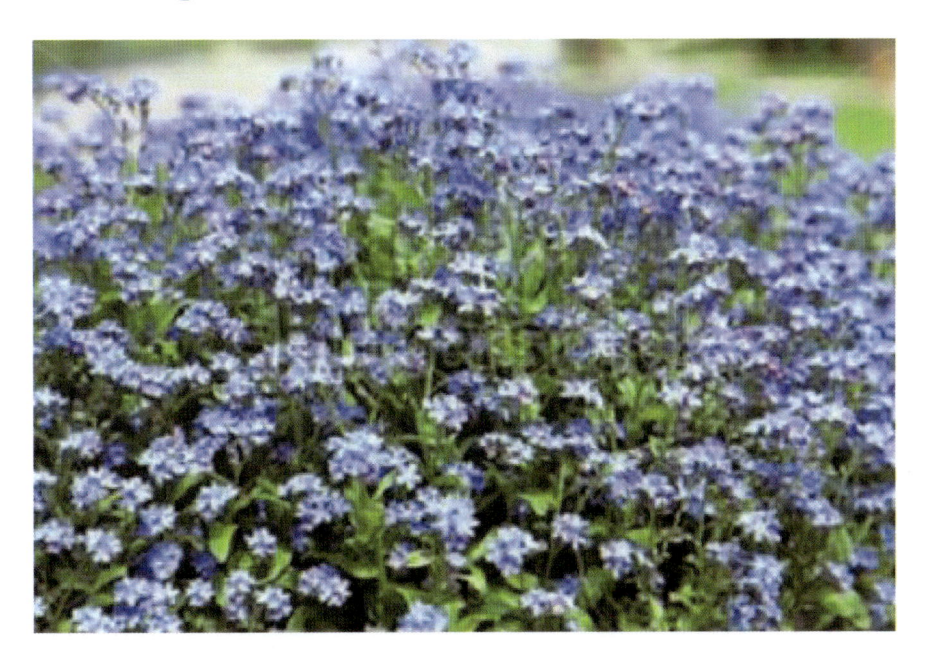

Keywords: reveller, focus, insights, reveal, hidden, concealed, access, dreams

Indications: Solar plexus, heart chakra, 3rd eye
For the deeply hidden buried stuff that is difficult to access.
It has a lightening and settling effect on the heart chakra.
It helps with dreams and visions to understand and remember them.
Helps to pay attention to details and helps with focusing the mind .

Healing Qualities: This delightful essence, took ages before it revealed its secrets. At first I used to see flashes of Blue, I heard giggling.
Gradually the journey started to unfold, at the time keeping information hidden it was so obvious. It was all about

revealing.

This beautiful little flower essence is for finding things out, questing. It is for things that are hidden Away in the darkness of our being that we have really buried. Which frees us up.
It helps with our dreams and visions helping us pay attention to detail, and helps with memory recall
It lightens and settles the heart. There is a childlike quality about this essence. It helps to access the Fairy realm.
This is a gentle but strong essence, and give power within.

Notes: The essence has a child like quality, bringing with it a childlike quality. It helps to access the fairy Realm.

Forsythia

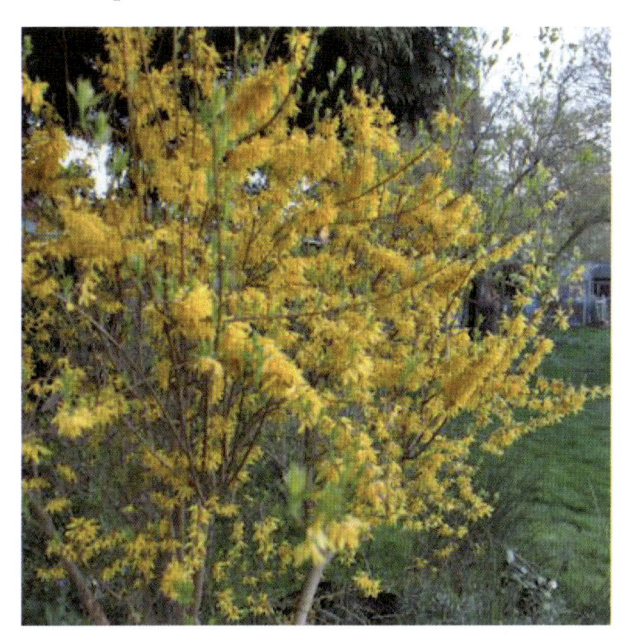

Keywords: ancestral, pattern breaker, deep sadness, desolation, courage, addictions, direction, fear

Indications: This essence is about 'Being who you are' Helping you with what you need to do in life without being affected by the fearfulness or negative emotions and actions of others.
It helps clear old patterns of behaviours.

Healing Qualities: It helps to remain alert aware, but strong and fearless to your core.
Helping you to steer your own course. Making your own decisions and explorations. Thinking and acting outside the box.

Notes: *Jan Rose's*
Strong almost painful feel in left hand. Firm hold. Heart.

Flat land gridded with canals. Symmetry and man made order in the middle of nature. Lots of activity within this enclave, much busyness. High fence rings this vast watery metropolis. Bare land from the fence to the base of the mountains. Long horned mountain goat watches from the base of a mountain. Bounds across the no-mans-land and leaps the high fence bordering the settlement. Explores with interest, trotting around looking at everything.

People back away, terrified of this inquisitive intruder. Arm themselves with big sticks and oars and run down the straight lines of the canals to try to attack him. The goat dodges nimbly this way and that, bounding over waterways and across any obstacles, completely perplexing his pursuers.

He always remains alert and one jump ahead of the mob, but still manages to see what he wants to see and explore their territory. He is aware of their intentions but not in fear of them. He examines and explores with interest without allowing the fearful and aggressive hordes to disrupt or interfere with him.

When he has seen all that he came to see, he nonchalantly hops onto the roof of a boat and uses it as a springboard back over the fence. Once over, he turns to face the still overexcited noisy crowd on the other side. Even after he has calmly moved out of their view, the people are still jittery and nervous, peering through the fence in dread in case he has returned.

Foxglove (pink)

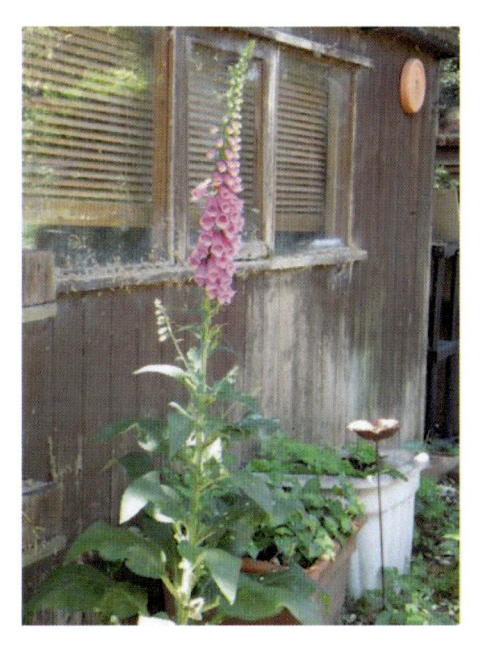

Keywords: confusion, clarity, heart, perspective, manifesting

Indications: Clears the head, heart healer,

Healing Qualities: this beautiful pink foxglove really communicated that it wanted to be created into an essence. It certainly lifted my heart, I could feel warmth in my heart. It help put things in perspective. It seemed to wrap itself around you bringing you into alignment.

its about bringing into being what is needed into our lives. It will also help to speak our highest truth.

Gingko-Biloba

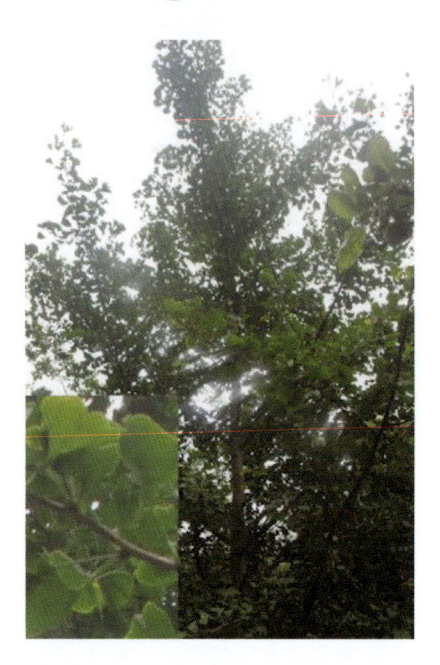

Keywords: regroup, move on, release, hold space, clarity, emotional, mental bodies, harmonises, interdimensional, ancestral, peace, conflict

Indications: congested thinking, confusion, can't see wood for the trees. Helping to release and let go. Harmonises emotional and mental bodies.

Healing Qualities: Where conflict or you may be conflicted it helps to regroup and move on, enabling to let go and be released. When this essence was being birthed I was experiencing conflict it helped me move on.

Helen ward insights, this is an inter-dimensional essence, lifting various veils that have remained hidden. There is a connection with the mystery of life and how life begins again within each of us. How we find the ability to regroup and move on. Helen experienced the magical realm

Notes: the Ginkgo tree first appeared 290 million years ago, which makes it one of the oldest species in the world. It is sometimes known as a "living fossil" it originated from China and Japan. The oldest ginkgo was planted in the 1760. at one stage it nearly became extinct but people helped it to survive. It is often associated with health and wellbeing. Said to help with the memory.

Hazel Catkin

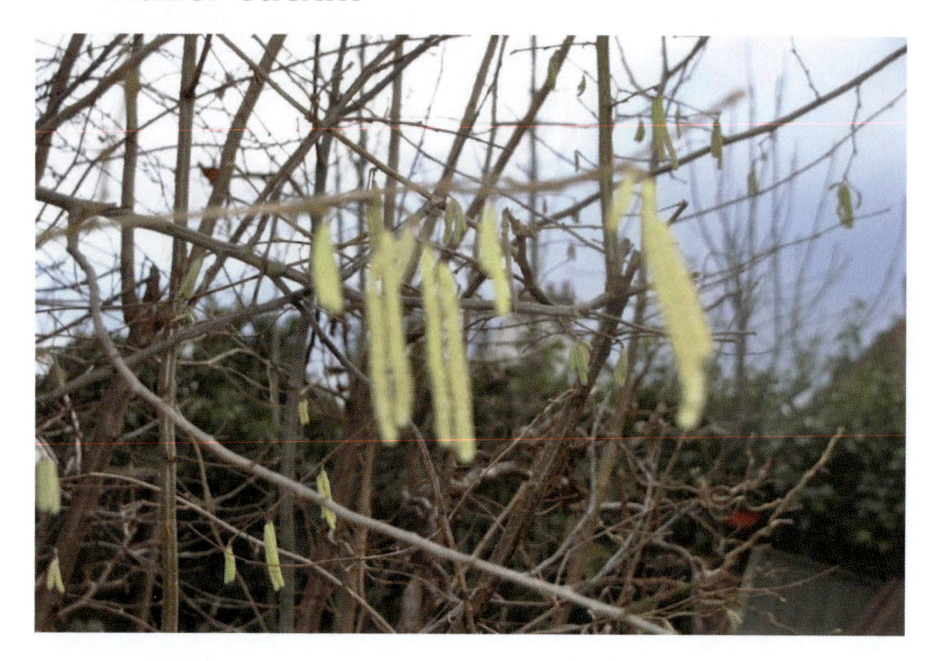

Keywords: freedom, confidence, self doubt, focus, decision, torment, confusion, conflict

Indications: Tying ourselves up in knots.
It releases us from torment. This essence is about flying free. For when we panic. "Can I" "can't I" "will I won't I" "No I can't" Tying ourselves up in knots.

Healing Qualities: Hazel Catkin can help us when we go into a state of no focus.
We swing in our decision making not able to commit with confidence. This essence can help to settle this state down.
The Hazel I made this essence from is a 'Twisted Hazel' so, this came as no surprise as to what states it can help with.
it will often come up with clients who freeze in this state with their indecision and has proved itself to be really effective giving them confidence with their decision making.

Hibiscus

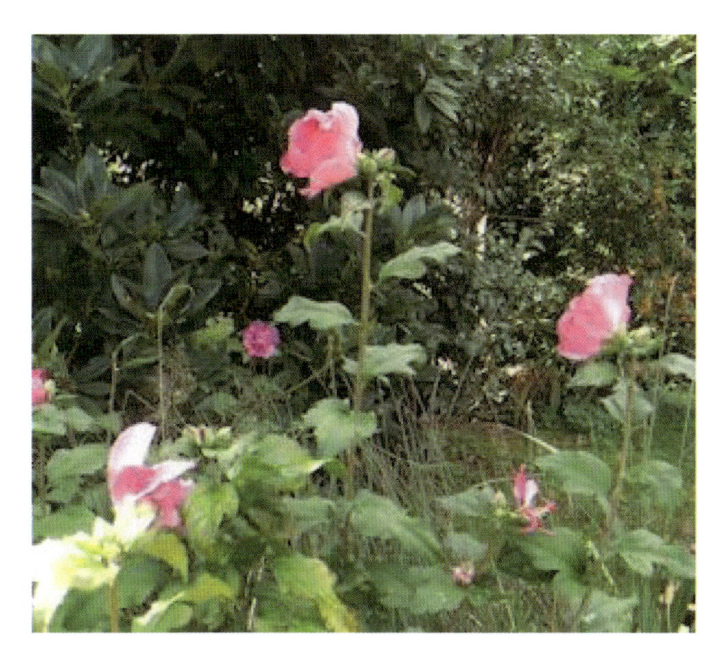

Keywords: uptight, calms, energy, settles, chi, relaxation

Indications: ears, solar plexus, heart chakra is indicated, It works on the chi, prana. Settles things down.

Healing Qualities: sooths and settles down the core, helps to quieten things down.
It helps when we are up-tight, bringing feelings of relaxation.

Holly

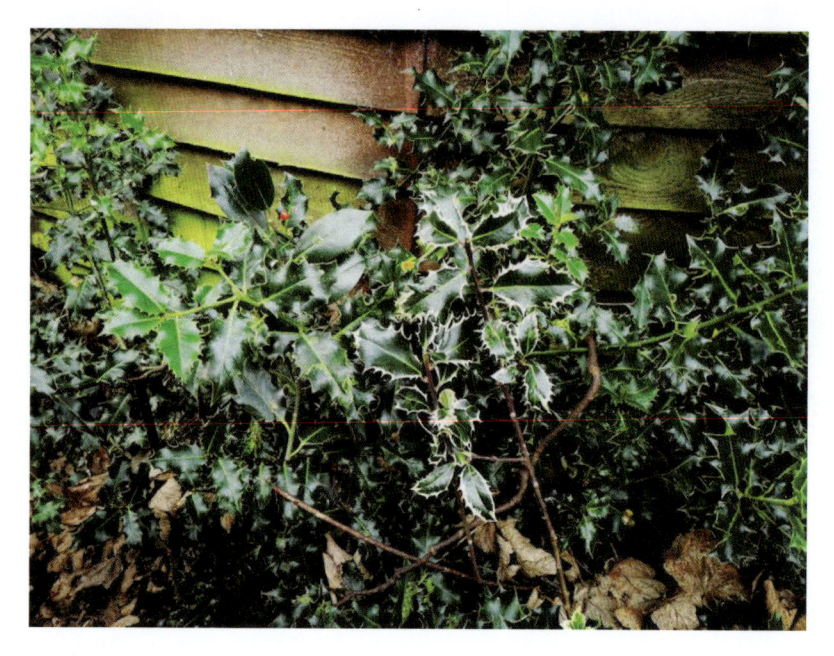

Keywords: compassion, harmony, meditative, love, understanding, protection, anger, aggression, fear, jealousy, revenge, resentment, irritation,,heart, self-love

Indications: heart chakra, access a positive attitude. Helps engender feeling of love to the self and others.

Healing Qualities: This is also one of the Bach essences for jealousy, anger, rivalry. The lyrics that came into my head were "we are circling, circling together, singing, singing my heart song" (we are circling. Written by Buffy Sainte-Marie)

This essence was created from 2 different hollies, on a full moon in Gemini, as this essence was being created I heard blackbirds singing and saw 4 blackbirds which really lifted my heart. It helps to be mindful of finding a different way, seeing things in a positive light.

it reaches through the mental debris and confusion of life to get access to our spiritual centre.

Notes: 12.12.19 in my garden full moon in Gemini

Honesty

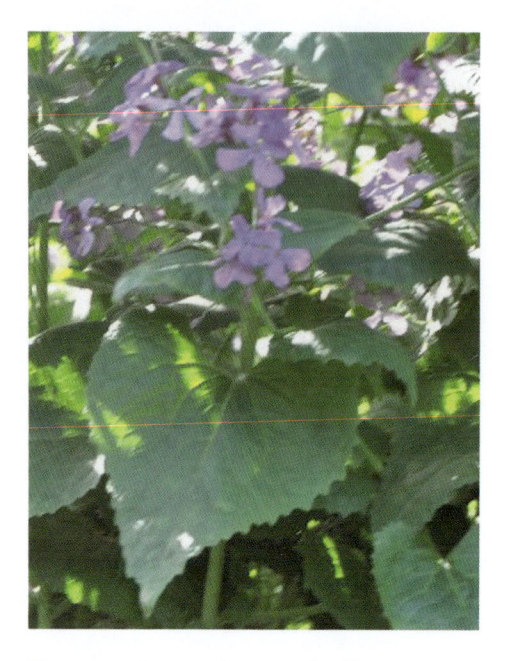

Keywords: truth, gut-feeling, empower, honesty

Indications: Heart chakra, solar plexus,
It is about Truth and self- honesty. Linking us into the Gut feelings. It helps to nurture, bringing in harmony with in the self. It also empowers.

Healing Qualities: this beautiful essence engenders the heart it helps with self-honesty, openness, and self-respect

Inipi Moss

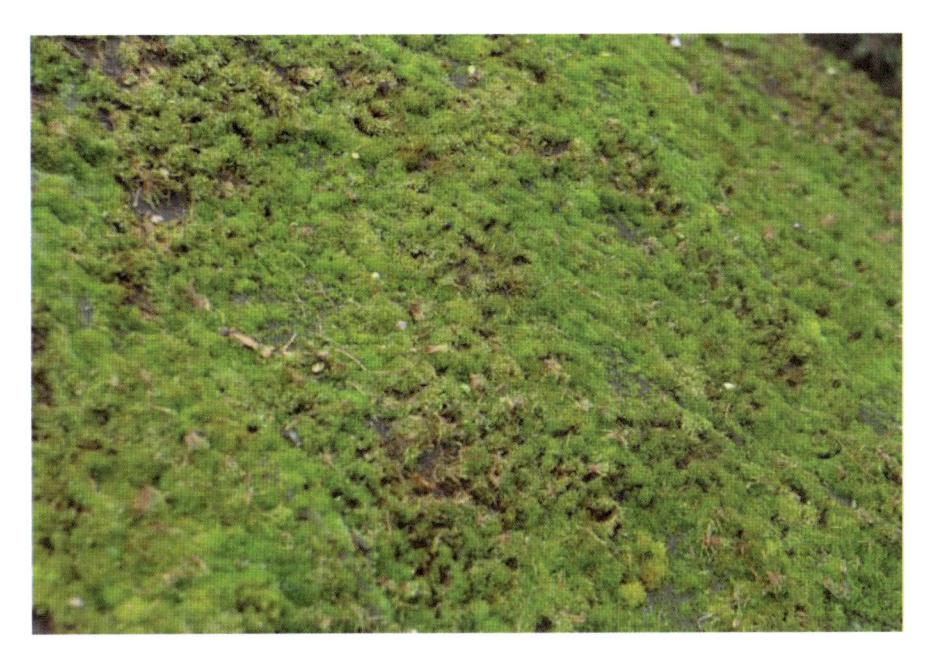

Keywords: fire balancer, balance, grounding, energiser, insights, filters, roots, rhythm

Indications: sacrum chakra. This beautiful deep very strong essence, helps to ground and helps us to get back to our roots. Fire element balancer.
Filters out the bad leaving with the good stuff.

Healing Qualities: This beautiful deep very strong essence, helps to ground and helps us to get back to our routes. It helps to rebalance, bringing us back to our own rhythm. It also helps to energise
Acting as a filter taking the good and the bad, leavening us with the good.
It is good for insights.
Jan Stewarts insights This is a fire element balancer. It is a strong grounding essence. It is about getting back to your routes.

Notes: This essence came about from sweat lodges that we have in our Garden. The moss grew on the structure we keep up. Overtime moss grew and developed. I knew I needed to make an essence out of this unique plant. Can be used in sweat lodges.

So, after an Imbolc sweat in 2015 the time had come. I pulled the moss away from the structure and left it to float on the water.

Japanese Azalea

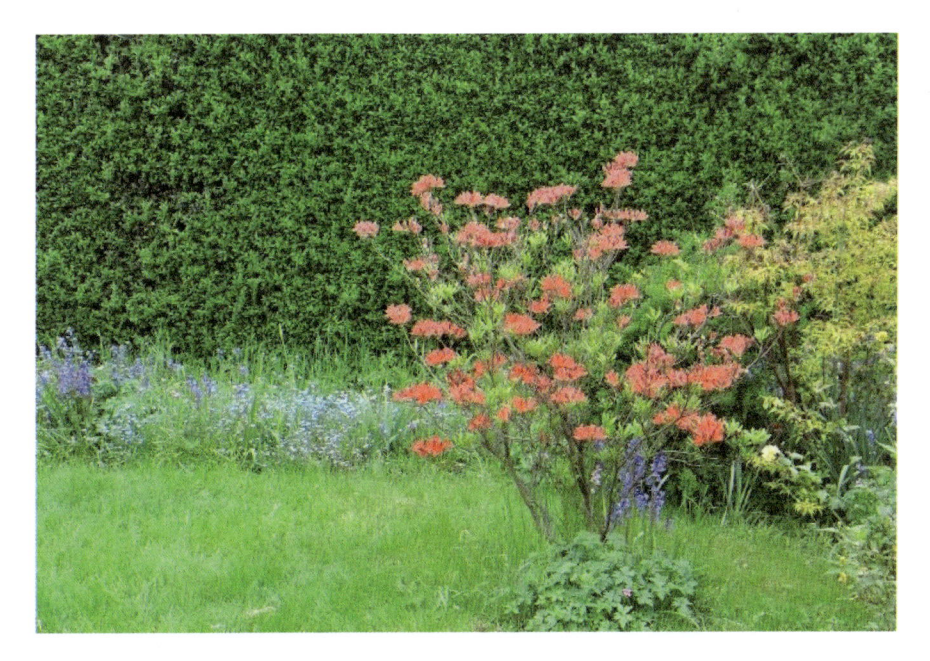

Keywords: energy, downloader, freedom, place, clarity, pattern breaker, mental anguish, battered, bruised by life, turmoil

Indications: 3rd eye chakra,
Taking on new forms: Finding where you truly belong. Helpful when you no longer fit in and need to change helping you to flourish.
When bruised by life and are left feeling raw.
Downloader of information, energiser.

Healing Qualities: This is a good essence that helps us to understand our thought processes, bringing clarity to the mind. It helps us to understand our thought processes. When we are stressed, or in mental turmoil, it will settle the mind down. Good when we have been left feeling battered and bruised by life.
Helps us take new direction.
It is a downloader. It deprogrammers helps to break patterns (DNA?)

Jan Rose's Insights:
This essence is all about taking on new forms. Finding the life that fits you and allows you to flourish. Useful for people who have tried out different professions and lifestyles but who don't feel they have quite found the one that fits them. Helpful when life has become stagnant and you no longer fit your situation, helping you to find where you now belong. Free yourself and you also free those around you.

Notes: *Jan Rose's Insights:*
Shadowy leaves, dark against a mustard yellow sky. Rustling and moving in the wind. The sound of rustling becomes overwhelming. The wind is becoming stronger and stronger, blowing leaves to the ground. Dark trees silhouetted against the mustard and white clouded sky. Dark leaves litter the ground.
The wind whips some of them up into the air, blowing them together to form the shape of a bear. (The way it was done reminded me of the starling marmiton). It lumbered around, turning its head until the wind disperses it. The leaves are reformed into a giant turtle/tortoise. It moves around slowly, looking about. The wind gives another almighty 'Whoosh' and disperses the shape, casting the leaves to the ground.
The wind gusts again, causing the leaves to rise and form an eagle. It flies around the sky and trees, wheeling and screeching, riding the thermals. It rises further and further up with the air currents and is taken away by the wind, its form complete, until it is just a small dark speck in the sky.
All is quiet and still. Gradually the mustard sky turns to blue, the dark silhouetted tree trunks become brown/grey with clearly textured bark. Green buds form on branches. Birds begin to sing and build nests. Life moves on.

Japanese Azalea (Saki)

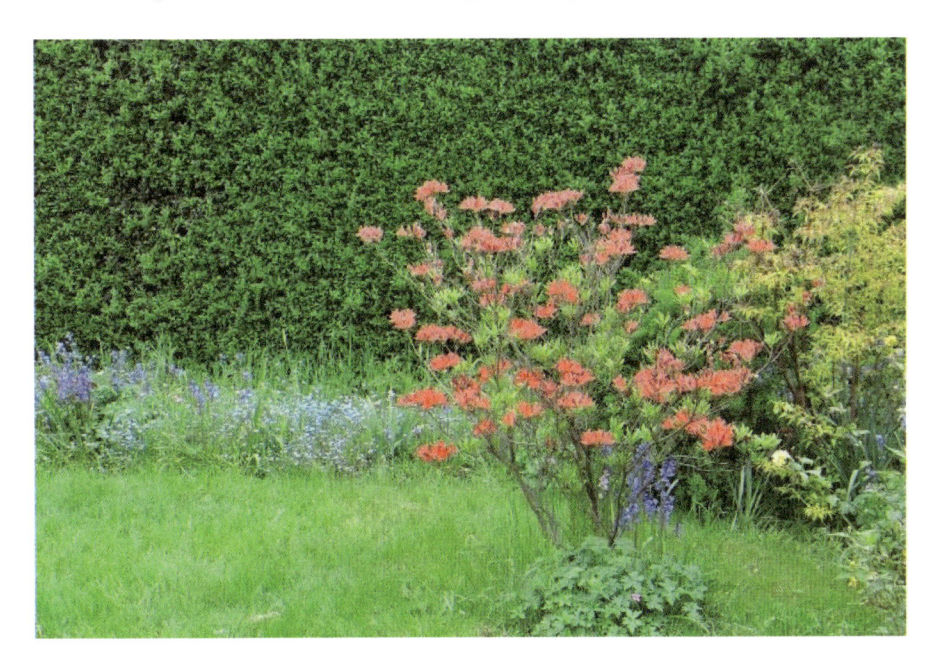

Keywords: clarity, balances, release,

Indications: 3rd Eye chakra. Chakra balancer.
All senses fully functioning.
Alert and aware of all incoming messages and information.
Works on the meridian system.
Pushes issues to the surface that need to be dealt with, to give clarity.
Releasing issues and emotions bring them to the surface to be dealt with.

Healing Qualities: This essence is a good 'opener' use this first, and then the original Japanese Azalea
This essence helps to clear stuff out, releasing what we are hanging onto. Brings issues and emotions to the surface to be cleared bringing clarity.

Good to take when out of sorts.

Notes: *Jan Roses insights*
Yellow parasol against a clear blue sky. Other parasols in other bright colours appear, leaving just snippets of sky visible.

Jan Rose gave the following description of her experience Throws out anything that is not needed or is detrimental. Releases in whatever way is needed e. g. Tears, speaking out. NB - I took this essence a couple of weeks after I had been involved in a car accident. The first day I felt incredibly tearful and wobbly. The next day I went for acupuncture to clear the shock and my body was throwing the needles back out as soon as they were put in to certain points. The acupuncturist had to rethink then placed them elsewhere and they stayed put. I cried throughout the entire session and was racked with tremors and twitching the whole time. I had a flash of inspiration about how I have always dealt with shock positively and negatively. Fine afterwards. Have never had needles do that before.

Kefalonia Bamboo

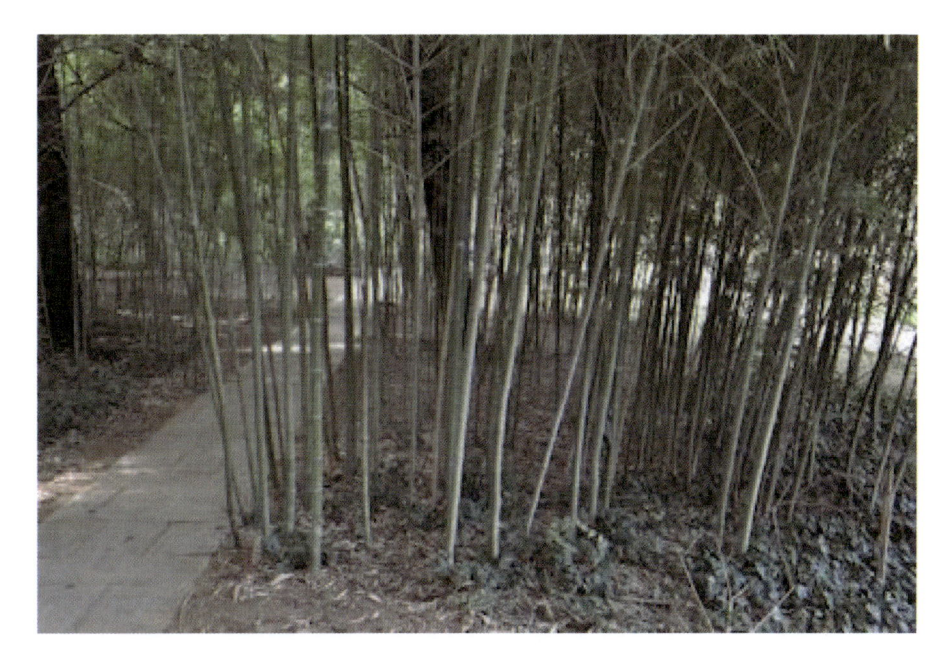

Keywords: strength, purpose, drive, cleanses

Indications: solar plexus chakra, sacrum chakra
It has a cleansing effect. Helps to drive one forward with purpose and determination.

Healing Qualities: This essence is all about strength, purpose, and drive. It gives you the drive to move forward, understanding the reason. It will give you the determination and understand the purpose .
When I first took this essence, I became very aware of my teeth.

Notes: with in the gesture of Bamboo there is certainly a lot of drive and determination to succeed with what it needs to do. There is much strength.
Bamboo is extraordinary. You can eat it, make cooking utensils, make a fire with it, make clothes with it, and live in a house made of it.

Kerria Japonica

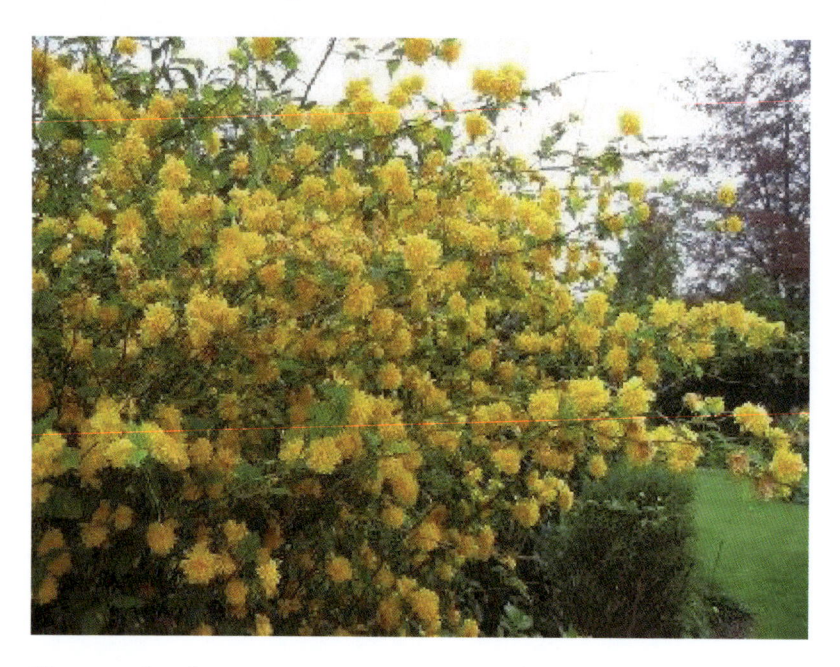

Keywords: harness, scatter, energy, release, emotions, action

Indications: heart chakra,
To contain and harness scattered energy, emotions. For scattered skittish energy

Healing Qualities: This essence is about dealing with emotions and problems as they arise, rather than leaving them until they become too big to be manageable. Releasing pent-up emotions and suppressed feelings. Taking the bull by the horns with timely and decisive action.
Holds the chambers of the heart chakra in peace and stillness while the turbulent emotions run through and clear.
It protects and grounds the heart chakra.

Notes: *Jan Rose's Insights*
China. Looking out from under a coolie hat at a blue hazed view of rice paddies and far off mountains. There is an older man, with grey

hair and a beard, also wearing a coolie hat. We are both looking out over the land. It is early morning, with people just arriving to work on the paddies.

The man points up to the sky. There is a cloud dragon forming and moving towards us over the sky. Slowly, unperceptively, it takes shape. It darkens to a deep shade of grey and becomes clearer and more detailed. It is very fierce looking. It gathers towards it storm clouds from across the sky, then let's fly with a terrific storm. Thunder, lightning and torrential rain. People run for cover.

Gradually the storm abates. The sky clears, rain stops and sun shines. The dragon is smaller, made up of small white fluffy clouds. It is smiling and peaceful.

Ladies Mantle

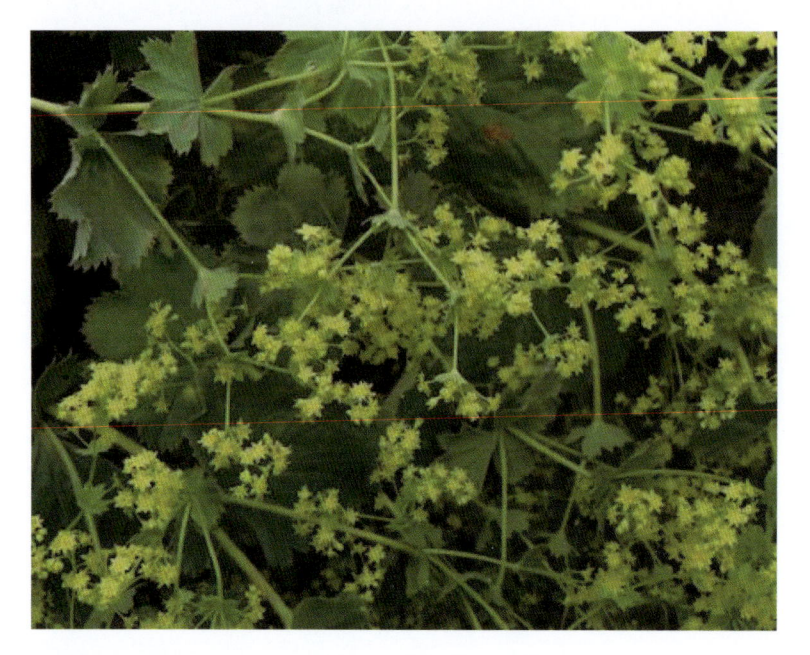

Keywords: pattern breaker, cleanse, empower, protection, purpose, self destruction, purpose, addictions

Indications: Helps with heart chakra challenges. An essence for the feminine. Breaking our patterns . Brings us to our true purpose.

Healing Qualities: Brings us back to stand in our power. Restore you back to your true purpose.
Helping us to break with patterns of self destruction.

Lambs Ears

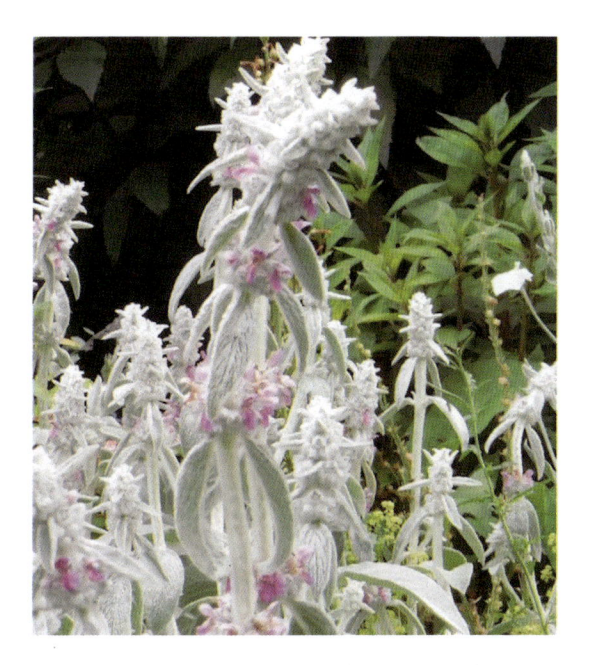

Keywords: focus, smooths, strength, peace, quietens chakras, purpose

Indications: This smooths the pathways and strengthens you to be clearer where you are going, keeping you on your path.
It helps keep the balance, and brings peace to you, despite the challenges.

Healing Qualities: Lambs ears are really smooths and velvety. This is an essence which is about smoothing the way, keeping you on track, despite challenges. When I made this essence. I was being side tracked with a challenging issue, despite this I was able to keep on track, keeping focused where I needed to be.

Laurel

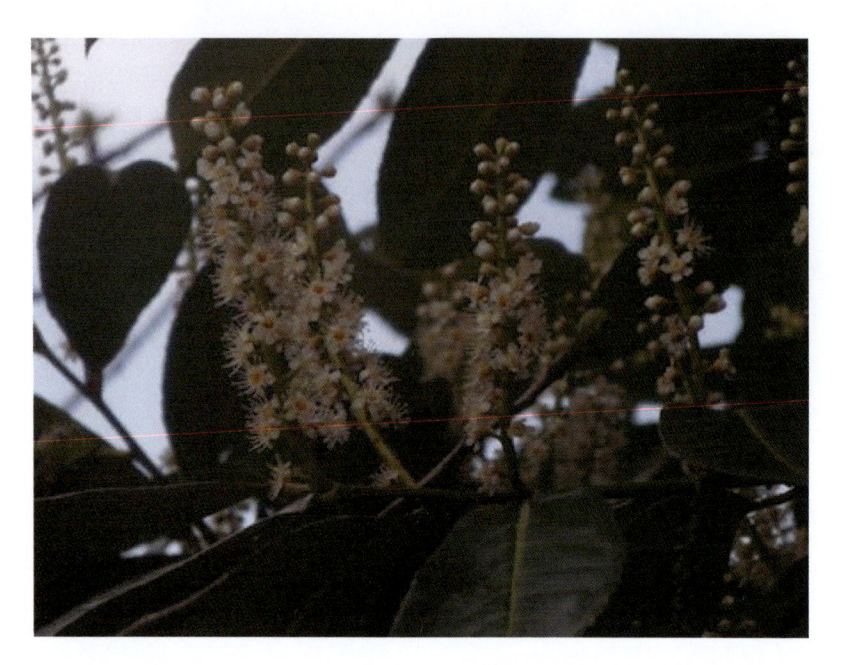

Keywords: success, confidence, strive, night terrors, psychic protection,

Indications: 3rd eye chakra & Crown chakra. This essence is all about success, and confidence. It helps us to strive.
It settles night terrors and is helpful with psychic attack.

Healing Qualities: When I made this essence, I was having some issues with confidence, and so the gift from the Laurel came to help.

Jan Rose's Insights
Helpful with, Psychic attack, ET when asleep or unconscious. May be good when someone is in a coma to give protection when out of the body on the astral realms.
Helping you to 'keep your head in volatile or crucial situations.

In the gesture we look at the Laurel, all throughout it remains strong, unyielding, unaffected by outer conditions or changes around it. An indication of its strength and the protection it provides.

Notes: Made from laurel leaves and berries. Snap shots in different lights and weather conditions; the Laurel remains the same. Combines well with Viburnum Burkwoodii

Lotus

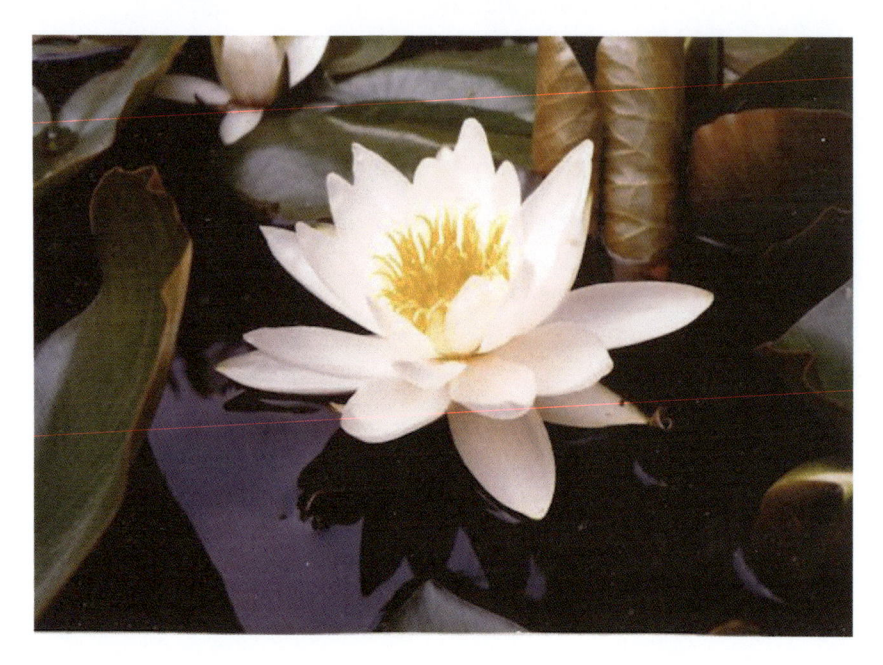

Keywords: expansive, insight, visions, power, clarity, flow, insight

Indications: crown chakra, 3rd eye chakra, throat chakra,
Expansive, with insights, really good to take before for vision quests, giving us deeper insights.
Takes one into self- love vibration. For digging deep, like into the roots of things

Healing Qualities: This essence helps things to flow, it helps us to dig deeper gaining deeper insight into ourselves. It helps us to see things in a different way.
Give us insights into different realms, taking you into different levels. It brings with it clarity to the mind.

The Lotus grows in the Mud. The deeper and thicker the mud the more beautiful the flower. This essence is all about insights and visions into other realms and realities.

Jan Rose's insights
Good before vision quests or journeys. You will learn about other realities and dimensions but also gain deeper insights into yourself and your soul's progression as it makes its way through time.
It expands our awareness, on many levels.

Notes: *Jan Rose's Insights:*
Mirage in a deep blue sky of a Middle Eastern city. Buildings, carts, people, animals all clearly visible. Lots of hustle and bustle as they all carry on about their daily business. No sound.
This is not a delusion - it is a vision of an actual city and its people and its daily happenings, just in another time or dimension to ours. They all exist, but just not here. We are being offered a glimpse Very, very powerful stuff - use with care!!
Into what lies beyond our own existences and experiences. Just because it is not physically tangible here does not mean to say that it does not exist at all.
(The tingling in my hand continued for a very long time after the bottle was put down)

Mahonia

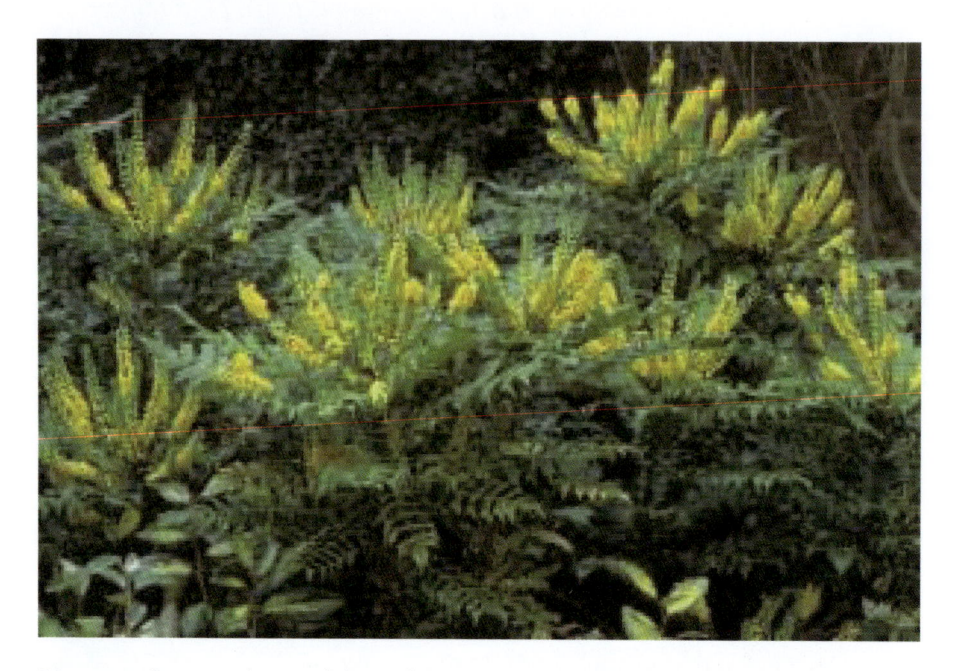

Keywords: warrior, spirit, quietens, peace, strength, fortitude, self-knowledge, discipline, courage, self-reliance, anger, self-control, fear, intimidate, power, intimidated, ancestral, anger

Indications: Heart chakra, Solar plexus chakra, Strong heart chakra, Brings in warrior spirit. Useful in intimidating situations. Brings peace, Strength Self-control. Useful for anger, helping to connect you with your own power. Lifts the spirit.
Very male/masculine feel.

Healing Qualities: Useful when you find yourself in intimidating situations where you may end up by being too passive or too aggressive just from sheer nerves. Feeling your own power and being able to use it in an assertive and effective way.
It is useful with Ancestral healing. Particularly where we need to stand up for ourselves against, family structures and systems.
It brings emotional healing and balance. It is also useful for issues with Anger.

It is uplifting to the spirit.
Clears fear from the past.

Notes: See a warrior tribesman, standing his ground. Not aggressive or threatening, but fully capable of using the right amount of force if needs be. Earthed and grounded. Ready for all eventualities. Perfectly attuned to his environment, constantly aware of his situation. Strong protective spirit around him. (Samoan?)

Mandrake

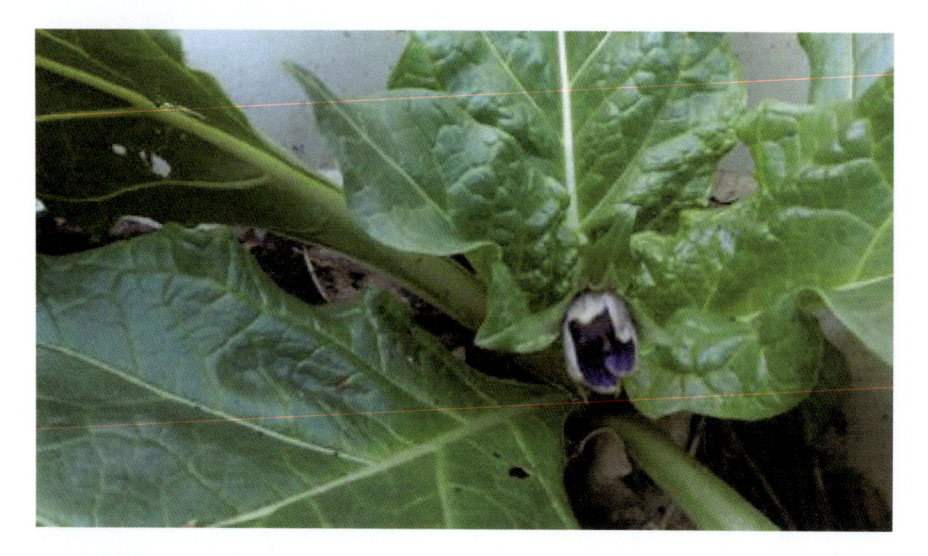

Keywords: activator, anchor, grounding, boundaries, clarifies, self determination, stabilise, strength, resistant, courage, express, straight talking

Indications: 3rd eye chakra, Heart chakra, Base chakra
Good effective boundaries. Clearing and clarifying our thought processes, it can help to speak your truth in a calm and effective manner.
Brings with it bravery and an unstoppable 'can do attitude' on different levels.
This essence empowers other essences and combinations, and unlocks hidden dimensions.
Reinstates boundaries, pathways and leys.

Healing Qualities: An experience I had with this essence was when a group of us sat with this essence. I sat with the essence calmly telling my truth about an issue that I was having at the time. This would normally have been difficult. However I remained calm and focused.

It is an essence that is strongly earthed and grounding, providing a solid base for upward growth and movement.

Jan Rose's insights

Helpful for talented but ungrounded people who cannot access their gifts or stick with a course of action or project until completion. This helps with change on a practical level.

With speaking our truth, enabling us to move things practically that have been difficult.

This essence is particularly helpful when engaged in magical activities or interacting with other realms.

Activating and accessing all senses, gifts, and innate talents.

Notes: *Jan Roses insights*
Cold yet tingling in the Hand. Magician Tarot,

Medlar

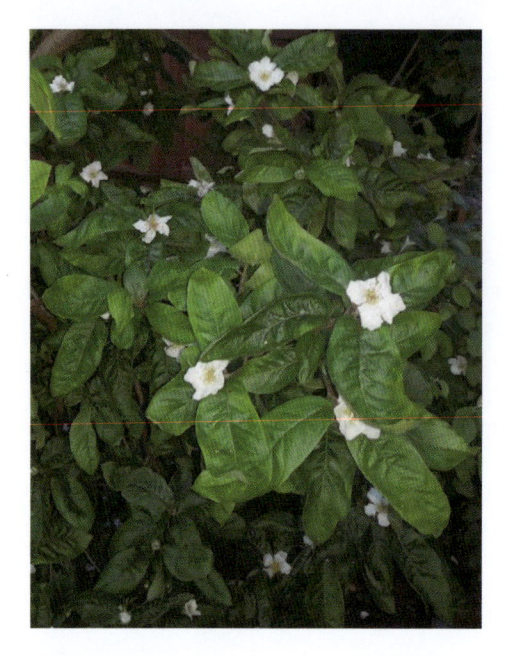

Keywords: interference, meddling, interfere, brightness of spirit, humour, openness, releases, stuck

Indications: lifts the spirit. Brings in openness embracing life.

Healing Qualities: where we are stuck in situations that are way outdated. This essence brings with it motivation and energy to achieve goals, giving you positive drive.

Mimulus

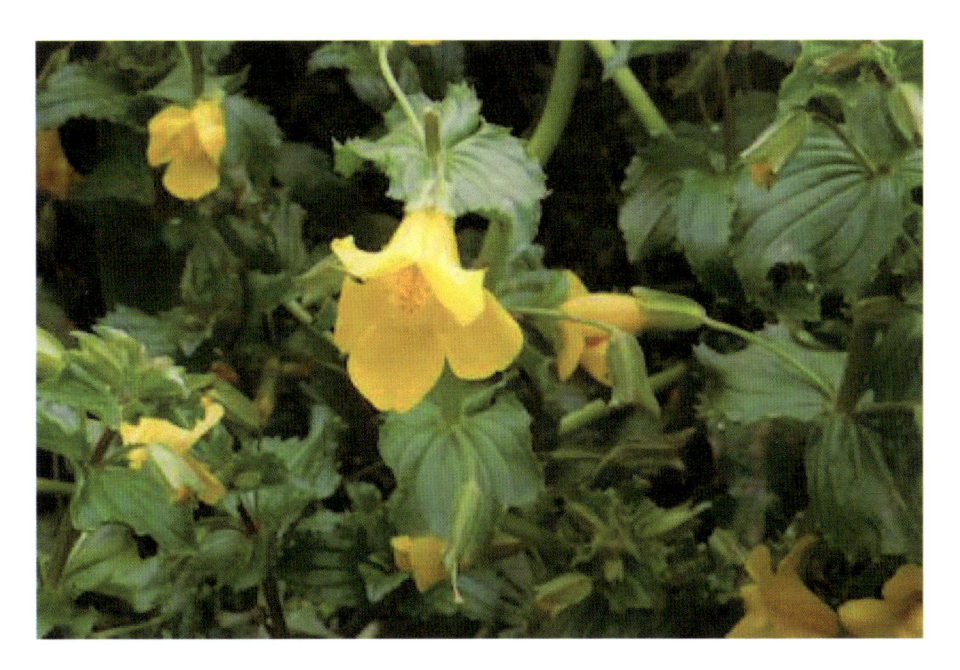

Keywords: fear, anxiety, safe, confidence

Indications: Throat chakra
This essence washes away fears and anxieties when we have been challenged by stressful situations that have emotionally unsettled. This essence has an energetic flow, moving things on.

Healing Qualities: This essence has an energetic flow, moving things on. It sparkles in the hand.
This is an essence all about confidence, to live your life happily and whole heartedly, without fear of judgement.
It helps us to easily connect to spirit, aware of synchronicities and blessings put there especially for you.
Jan Rose's insights
Safe and secure helps to link into the magic in life and flowing with it. Helps to remain undistracted by other's negativity, just easily and cheerfully getting on with ones own life and skipping unhindered along one's own path.

Notes: *Jan Roses insights*
As I worked with this I could hear Cheerful whistling.

Money Plant

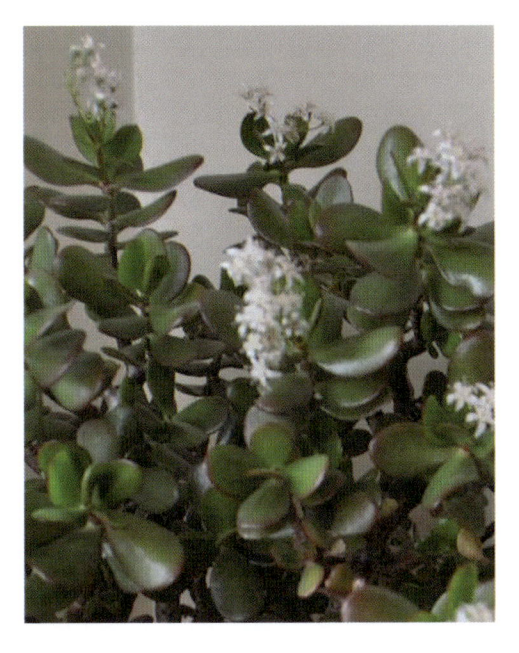

Keywords: energy, balances, calmness, soothes, alignment, harmonisation, abundance, manifests

Indications: Helps give and receive good things in life. Ears Turn the focus from the outer to the inner. Soothing effect on the emotions settling you down.

Healing Qualities: This essence is all about bringing yourself into alignment. Balance.
Preparation to give and receive the good things in life. Without these, true abundance and contentment are impossible.

Notes: *Jan Rose's insights*
Sunset - a pink and yellow streaked sky. Gentle sea reflects the colours above. Looking out of the mouth of a cave, paddling in the ocean, looking out towards the sunset. A naked man and woman are standing together in the sea, holding hands looking out at the sunset. Perfectly at peace, in harmony with themselves, each other and

nature. Sound of the sea/or when you place a shell to your ear. Temples.
Ears. Hands placed gently over ears. Eyes shut.

Montbretia

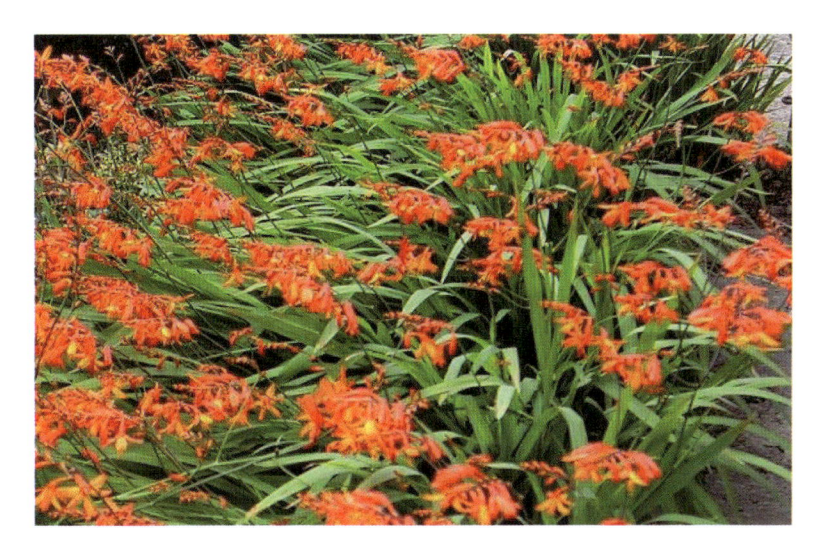

Keywords: fear, confidence, decisions, upheaval, release, peace, cleanse, land, battered, self sacrifice, regenerate

Indications: Brings balance and helps us weigh things up.
about confidence in decisions made
Brings peace after upheaval.
Good to use for traumatised land too.

Healing Qualities: Releasing old patterns of self-sacrifice. It, releases old emotional patterns tied into the past. It cleanses and promotes confidence. It brings balance and helps us weigh things up.

For major upheavals and life changes where your personal landscape is changing permanently and irrevocably, helping you weather and understand this and to rebuild and regenerate, in a different but better form for you.
When life's challenges have left us feeling raw and battered.

Notes: As I made this essence I was full of fear the whole time it was being energised. I felt nauseated which got worse. The fear and anxiety lifted once the essence was completed.

At the time I was dealing with a decision of whether to attend a gathering for various reasons I had decided not to attend.

Jan Rose's insights
Instability, Earthquake. Ground shuddering and cracking open. Fires in cracks. Dark dust forming in sky Alarmed birds and animal calls people trying to flee. Rely on instinct to get out of the way of danger- fast. Getting away from urban areas onto higher ground; a green hillside overlooking the city.
Ground moving huge cracks and still moving, but safer. Lie down flat on the grass and feel the earth's movements. Listen to the creaks, groans, and rumbles within the ground. Face down on the grass, feeling and hearing the earth: very primal. Eventually the tremors subside.
Get up and look around; still slight tremors and noises but gradually lessening. Look downhill buildings and roads swallowed up, great gaping holes in the ground, water erupting from the burst pipes, small fires. It is very different landscape and altered place from the upheaval.

Some years later: there are Blue clear skies, and eagle swooping and calling above. Looking down on the few broken buildings left there are birds flying in and out of their broken windows and doorways. Horses moving through the green vegetation that was once streets and small gardens. Wild Boar. Craters are now giant water pits, heron at the side. Vegetation abounds. A whole new world has risen from the shattered remains.

Nettle

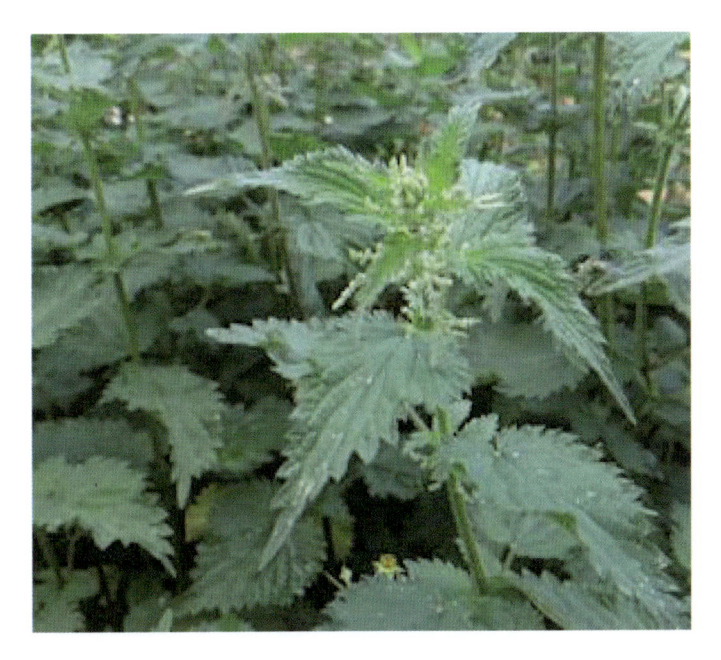

Keywords: connections, relationships, patience, anger, rage, old hurts, conflicts

Indications: Helps to take the sting out of conflicts within relationships. Sooths away anger and detoxes on an emotional level. It will help dissipate those intense issues that may have been embedded, releasing you. Helps protect and strengthens the energy field when affected by computers phones and other electrical interference.

Healing Qualities: This essence is all about accepting that situations, conflicts will take the time they take to resolve. It also helps make connections, which has been really apparent when included in combinations for clients. It seems to target a specific problem that is causing issues, tailored for them.

Acts as a protection with computers and electrical appliances.

New Zealand Flax

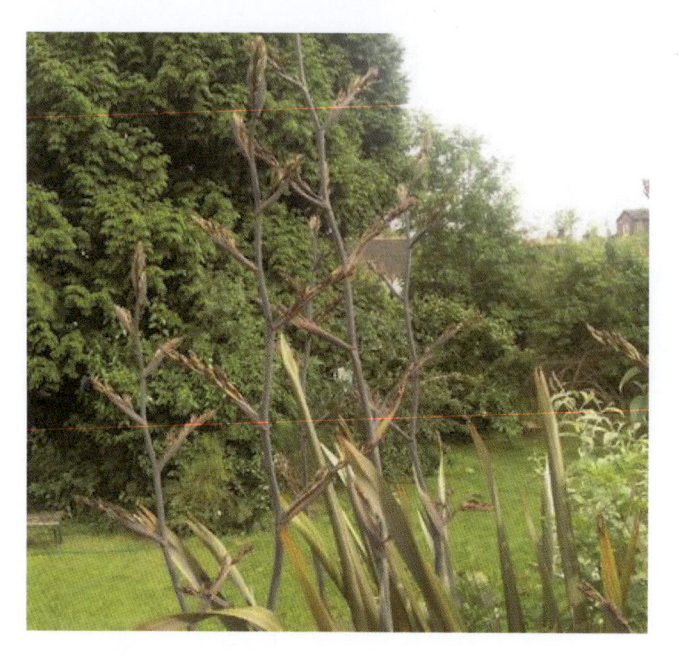

Keywords: peace, forgiveness, letting go, realigns, release, reintegration,

Indications: throat chakra, heart.
It brings a sense of peace, forgiveness, helping letting go,
Jan Rose's insights Central Governing Line meridian (from base of skull, up over head and down front of face to chin).

'When there is peace in the heart, all things are achievable'.
'Forgiveness brings a peaceful heart and tranquil mind'.
'Bringing stuff together. Basket weaving. Re-aligning'. It is also a good net worker

Healing Qualities: This amazing essence releases
Gentle, benign, non-verbal communication. Some things are too important to attempt to resolve with mere words. Heart to heart communication is key. Speech can be misconstrued and words misinterpreted , the heart cannot.

This essence takes us through a process, forgiveness letting go of resentment, releasing. Bringing a sense of peace. When we have peace in our Hearts we have tranquillity and all things are achievable.
When Jan Rose worked with this essence there was lots of yawning and releasing.

Notes: *Jan Rose's insights,*
when Jan linked in with New Zealand Flax, there was lots of yawning and releasing.
Yellow. Buddha head, golden. Flower garland (pink, Red) around the neck.
candles.
The Buddha statue is moving and smiling around at everyone.

Rafe Nauen's insights
T Torbay Palm, this plant died in 2008 but unlike the Palm, the flax's leaves remained crisp and dry, no sign of rot. We cut away the dead leaves, abut left the root ball as we would have killed the rambling rose that grows in its leaves. Again two years later it was back in full glory. What astonished me was the length of time to show any signs of activity.

Orange Blossom

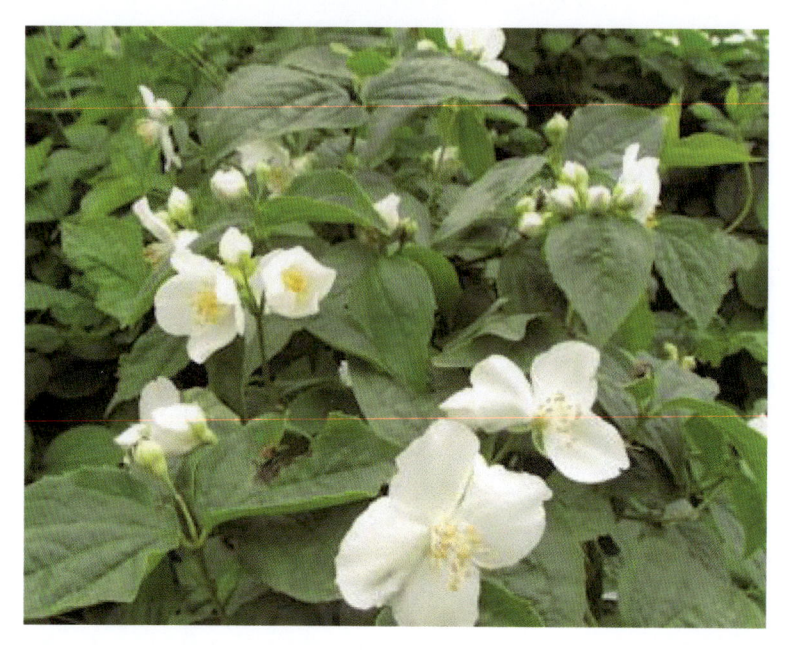

Keywords: adjust, peace, forgiveness, letting go, realign, release, reintegration, remembrance, authentic

Indications: Sacral chakra Base.
I have always referred to this as 'Trial by fire'
Helps to bring peace, helps to see what lies beneath the surface.
Taking control back. Being Authentic,
Helps to Harness our listening skills. When beset by trial helping us to overcome and not get dragged down

Healing Qualities: Helps to see the bigger picture bringing in remembrance. Protects you from the minutiae of life, and to remember what the situation was like prior to the problem arising This essence seems to have a lot to do with 'Seeing true'. Seeing what lies beneath the surface with people, places, situations. Perceiving other dimensions and realities. Seeing beyond the usual limited horizons that we are taught are 'normal'. The bigger picture.

All that is.
Good for seers and seekers.

Helpful when we are becoming caught up in the minutia of life and getting trapped by it. Helps us to see beyond our normal limits and horizons.

This essence is about self-love. Also, I think of it as an essence that deals with our trial by fire. Orange Blossom grows right by the fire pit and sweat lodge. It alters the way it flowers, stopping flowering the side by the fire and only flowering the side away from the fire. This essence is also about self-love.
Helps to gain control back. It is a good pick me up. It is also about learning to listen. It also enhances transferable skills. Helps to adjust the change that needs to take place.

Notes: *Jan Rose's Insights*

"I took it for 5 days when I went to Cornwall. I've had Chronic Fatigue, Exercise Induced Anaphylaxis, Asthma etc. for the past 5 years. The effect this essence had on me was all about 'Remembrance' – remembering what it felt like to be well and be myself again (the person beneath the medical conditions). To recover from a problem of long standing it is vital to be able to remember what it felt like to be yourself before it all happened – then you can start to reconnect with wellness.

: Jan describes the following journey.
Viewing film like images through the brow chakra. Above a darkened city at night, watching the lights of the cars below (USA?). Lights moving along the straight lines of the roads, orderly, conforming.
View expands beyond the city to the darkened hills/mountains. These grow in stature and intensity and dwarf the city until it appears as if in miniature. Lights and vehicles keep moving as before, seemingly unaware of what is around them.
Beneath the ground of the city, I can see the undulating form of the land, rivers and streams curving their way through. This image of

the land is transposed over the cityscape – 2 different realities juxtaposed.
City life continues, its inhabitants unaware of what is below and around them, seeing only their reality, their dimension, nothing more. The land is aware of all. The straight harsh lines of roads and blocks contrast sharply with the soft curves of the Earth.

Ox Eye Daisy

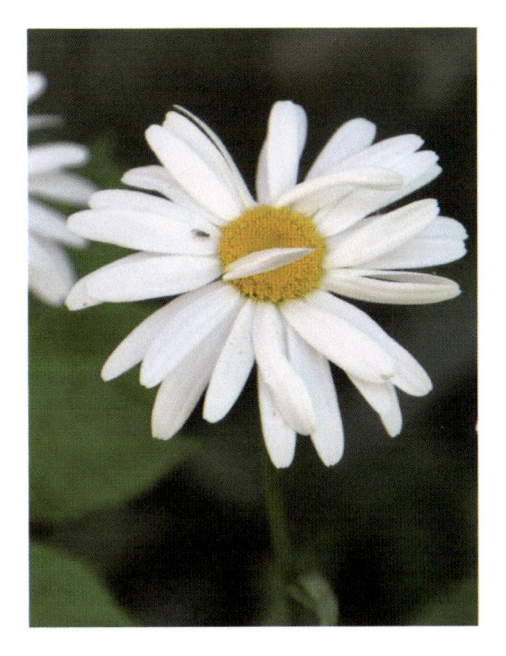

Keywords: un-complicate, clutter, clarifies, energy, youth,

Indications: Crown chakra, 3rd eye chakra, throat chakra,
This is an essence that will help with uncomplicating matters when the mind is clear life is less complicated. Taking us back to a time in life when life was less complex.

Healing Qualities: Recapturing innocence. The uncluttered mind. The essential core of being. Memories and how they shape who we think we are.
Simplicity and the perfection embodied within it.
Uncomplicating matters.
When we are being too complicated it will help to clear our heads. Taking us back to a place in our youth when things seemed far simpler.

Notes: *Jan Rose's insights:*

Young blond haired girl in strong sunshine (so powerful it is hard to make out many details). (A much younger female but very reminiscent of the one seen with the Pearl essence).
Calm and happy atmosphere. Little girl bare, sat playing in long grass that reaches her chest. Looks up at me, smiles and fades away into the sunshine.
Sound of the wind blowing through the long grass. Evocative, speaks of times past. Drops away. Sound of children singing nearby but can't see them through the brightness. Brilliant blue summer sky. Birds singing. Face of the little girl returns.

Peace Lily

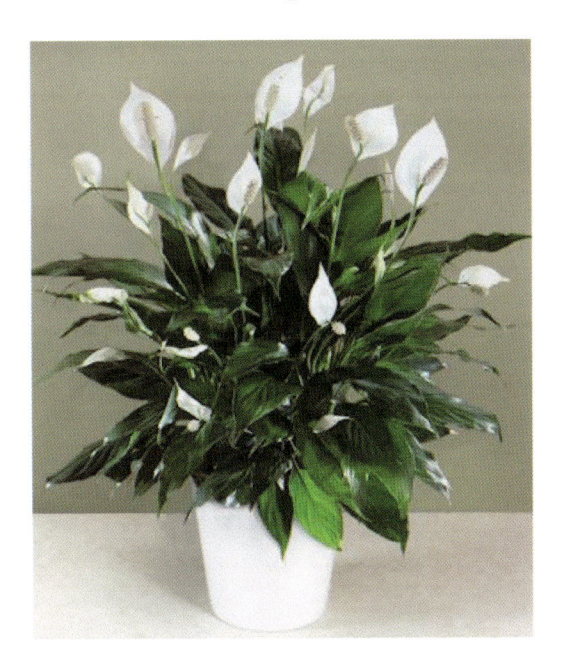

Keywords: forgiveness, resilience, release, geopathic stress, peace, chakras

Indications: Forgiveness and resilience are key with the Peace Lily. Geopathic stress is indicated. Helps bring us to a place of peace working on the mind, emotions and spirit, calming you down. Heart chakra is indicated.

Healing Qualities: As a Plant it is all giving.
Bringing calmness helping us let go It brings about forgiveness. It helps us to be resilient to the challenges life throws at us.
It also is about loving the self, helps us to reach out. The essence is like having a hug helps us to feel nurtured.
It brings about peace. Settles the mind, body, spirit and emotions.

A few years ago, I lost two Peace Lily's that were being neglected so putting them outside, I left them some time latter I noticed that they were putting shoots out. They are now back in the house quite happy thriving in fact!! This showed me so much about being resilient, forgiveness. Peace Lily's have always been one of my favourites.

Some years ago, I decided to repot all my peace lily's by the time I had finished I so many more these plants have loads of babies. So, after repotting. I decided to give them away to neighbours, friends and family. When I had done, I found out it was international peace week, coincidence? Plants teach in so many ways. We just need to be open to notice, and reflect.

Pear

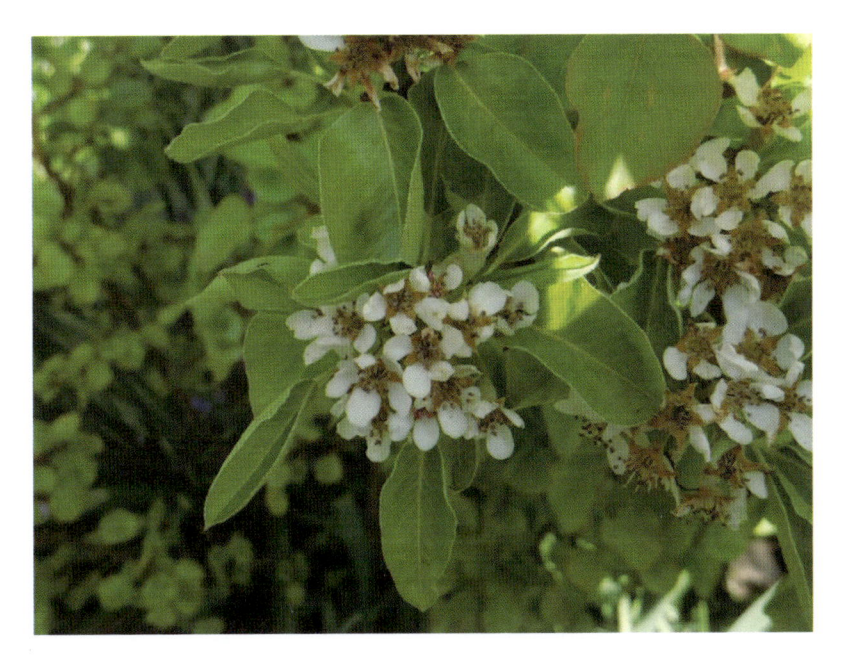

Keywords: peace, trauma, grief, integrates

Indications: lifts the spirit, integrating the mind body, emotional and spiritual bodies Major challenges and upsets.

Healing Qualities: this essence was birthed on the day I was at a dear friends funeral. When I decanted Pear essence it lifted my grief straight away.

Notes: this was birthed on the day of a dear friend's funeral

Peony

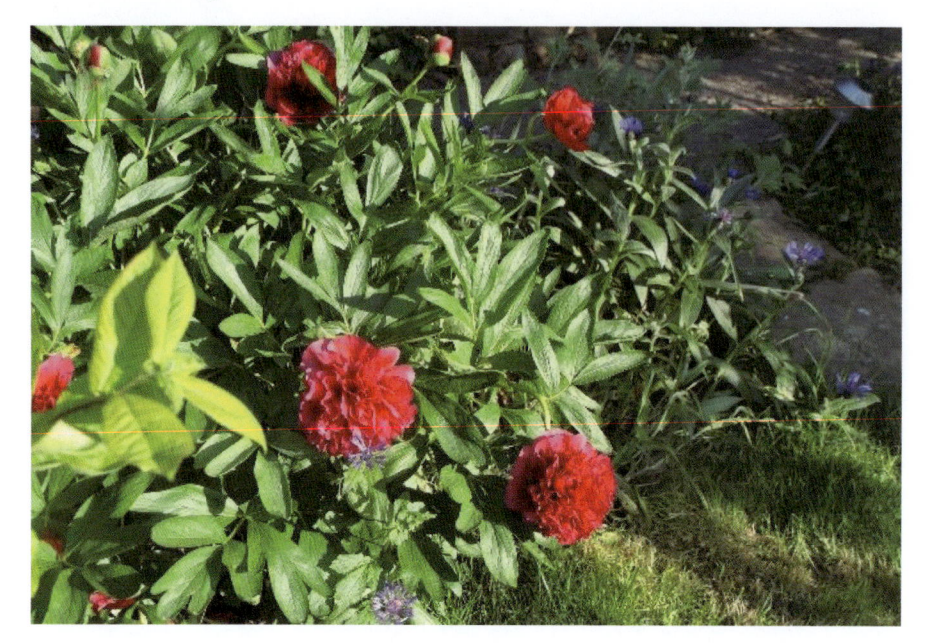

Keywords: revealer, compassion, gentleness, defences, resistant, release,

Indications: base chakra, heart chakra,
Reveals bringing out female qualities, for compassion and gentleness, for defences, for unfolding layers of the heart chakra. Where the heart has become closed. For use where feelings or attitudes are hardened and ingrained. Releasing with ease and grace, warm feelings, softening of any blows or hard edges.

Gently opening and reveals. This very feminine essence. Indicated for the base chakra. Combines well with white-pink Hawthorne. Good to use with the Dying
Would be good in a spray for a therapy room - helps clients to drop any defences and to soften and release.

Healing Qualities: It reveals helping us to realise by opening to others and the self, you will be able to put support in place. Would be good in a spray for a therapy room - helps clients to drop any defences and to soften and release.

Combines with White Pink Hawthorn

Jan Rose's insights
Where gentleness and compassion are needed. Can help with a person dying and the process. For driving one forward with awareness.
This very feminine essence. Indicated for the base chakra. Helps you to open up to others and to the self.

Pink Dog Rose

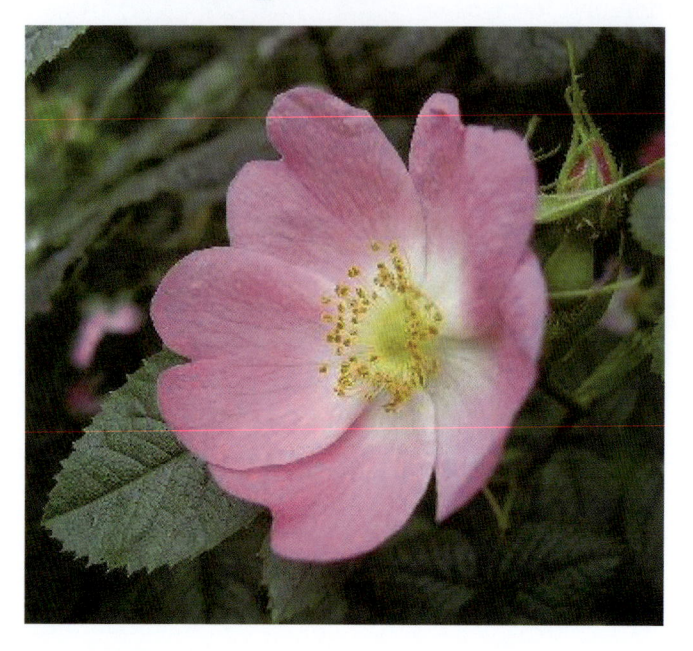

Keywords: balances, generosity, kindness, patience, heart, lungs

Indications: This essence balances the heart chakra it also helps to expand the energy of the lungs
It brings in the energy of generosity, kindness and patience, Its about loving the self and others. It expands the heart chakra, helping you to breath deeper with life.

Healing Qualities: When I first took this essence I felt the heart chakra expand. This is an essence to help heal the heart chakra.

Pink/White Hawthorn

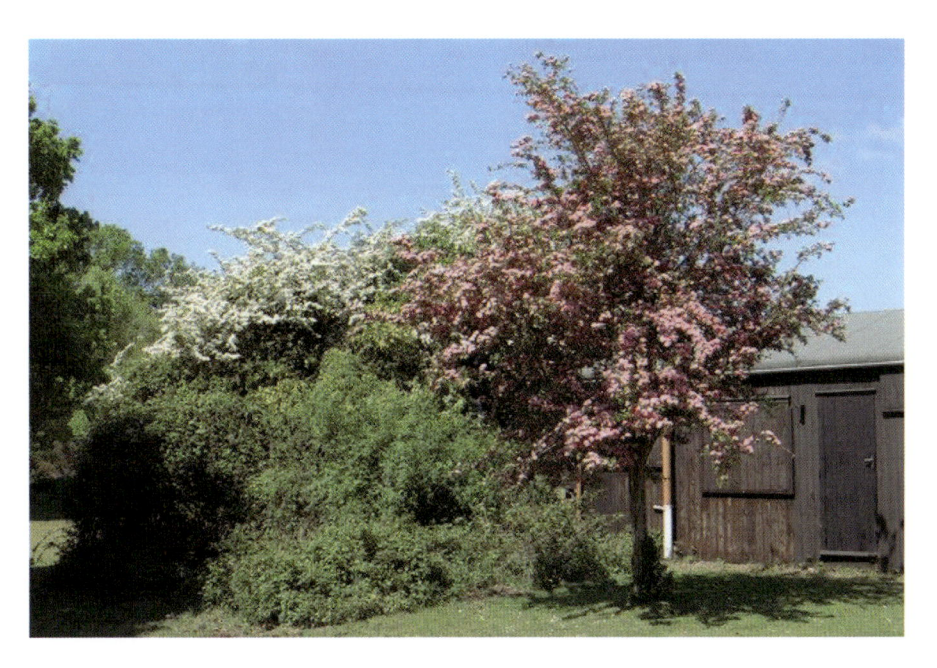

Keywords: heart warming, self love, empathy, ancestral healing, stress, aggression, divorce, custody battles, estranged family, heart

Indications: 3rd eye chakra, heart chakra,
'Love without fear' warms the heart chakra. It is learning to love the self. Softening of the heart and the World becomes a gentler place' It helps with nurturing yourself.
For aggressive damaged people or animals Would combine well with peony.

Healing Qualities: There is a tremendous warmth that is felt with this essence, it helps to feel softer and any fears are dissipated The insights Jan gives give us a really clear picture.

Jan Rose's Insights: This powerful essences teaches us to 'Love without Fear' feeling safe enough to feel. Giving us gentleness around the heart, it lightens the energy in this area, softening the

Heart.
For softening hardened, rigid attitudes, especially those passed down through family line.
Easing 'Heart-to-heart and emotional interactions with others, giving more empathy.

It can be used as a spray in ceremonies, so that all can participate with an open heart and be truly in touch with themselves, and their feelings and with others present.
Spray for difficult or emotional meetings e. g. Divorce, custody, estranged family former friends. Takes away the need to close or harden the heart to protect it, feeling safe and secure enough to dismantle your barriers. (Be good with the Limbic Reflexology, maybe sprayed on the hands or in the lotion as you work?)

Land, House- for bringing a heart into a place which has none e. g. Newbuild houses slammed up quickly and thoughtlessly.

Combines with Peony

Plum

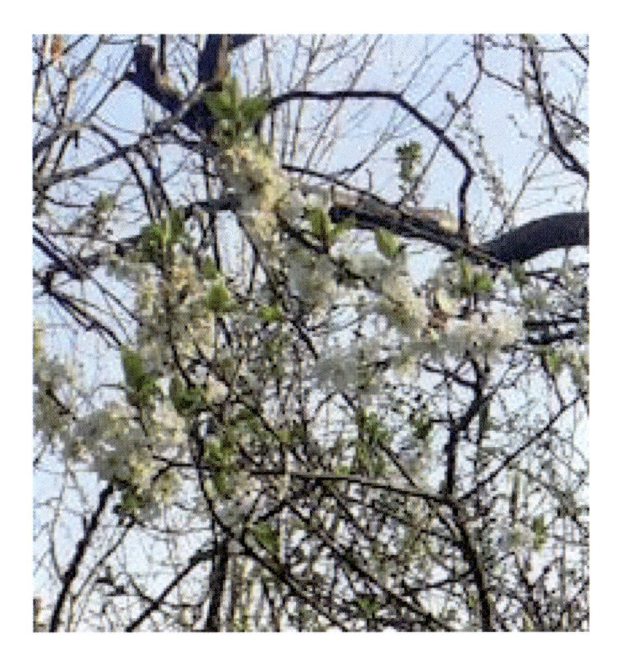

Keywords: adversity,

Indications: pushing through adversity, irrational thoughts and behaviour.

Healing Qualities: this was birthed from a dear old plum tree who has faced adversity and is still keeping going it still puts out its fruit. I associate this beautiful old plum tree with a dear friend of mine who was a tree surgeon who certainly had adversity in his life.

Pomegranate

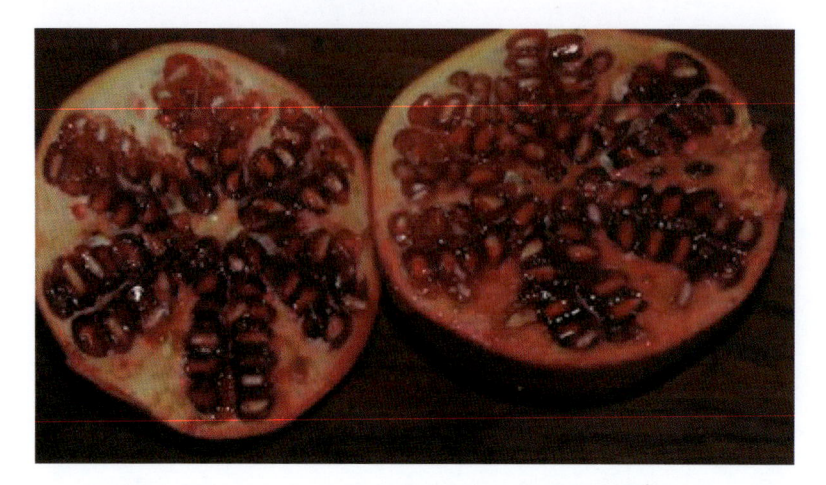

Keywords: anchor, inner tranquillity, chaos, lost soul parts, spirit, safe, strength, will, guidance, unsavoury, frazzled

Indications: when base, sacrum and solar plexus, chakras have been completely compromised through inappropriate contact. Holds you in a safe place.
Brings soul parts home. It strengthens the will.

This essence is a very spiritual essence working from a spiritual view. Helps people who are on a spiritual path.

Healing Qualities: Good when frazzled or overburdened with demands of life. Helps to find sanctuary of peace in your heart chakra and settles the thoughts amidst the chaos, the dark or unsavoury. This essence may help when there has been inappropriate contact and or touching.

It is indicated where soul parts have become detached, bringing back shattered parts of the self. It is an essence that will guide you through life. For those who walk a spiritual path.

Good when we need to look at our roles as parents and caregivers and realise that to nurture and care is natural, but there comes a point when it may inadvertently tip over to neurosis and control, which benefits neither parent or child, owner, or pet, carer or patient. Helps us to guide others being able to stand back and allow their journey to remain their own. It gives us the ability to bring plans to fruition but with a calm and light touch and understanding that everyone needs nurturing but also the space to grow.

Notes: When I made this essence, it was channelled and then I placed it into a pomegranate cut in half I left it there to ground it.

Jan Rose's Insights
Soft in the Hand but with a steady core strength. Centring, anchoring. I see a high priestess from the Waite, Colman Smith tarot pack. A strong assured but quiet woman, equally at home in both the physical and spirit realm. She knows how to nurture, but also how to give space to all that is waiting to be birthed, whether that is a child, idea, art, a garden or home, in fact anything that requires care but guidance with alight almost invisible touch. Acting as a quintessential at birth of the new, action, guidance in the comfortable silence.:

Red Flowering Currant

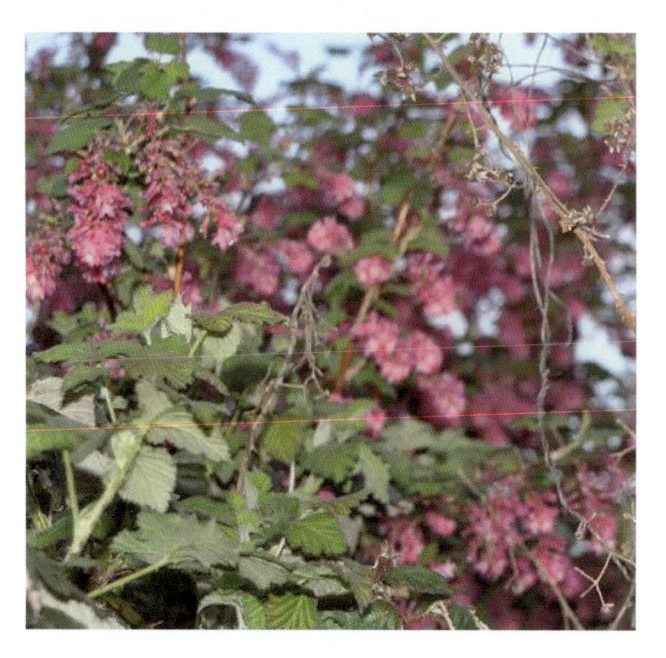

Keywords: feminine, cleanser, nurturing, cares hope, self worth, boundaries, tie cutting,

Indications: throat chakra, heart chakra.
Very feminine, heart chakra cleanser.
Good for carers, those with demanding partners, friends, family work or social colleagues. Living for the self not others. Reclaiming your life.
Learning to say NO and meaning it.

Decisive action for yourself without guilt. Knowing when to walk away.
Its about self nurturing regard for the self .

Healing Qualities: This essence is all about nurturing and hope.
It opens the mind, helps to seek the truth.
It is a cleanser and gives us a clean slate.

Jan Rose's insights Taking back your time and your life. Extricating yourself from draining people and or situations. Not allowing your time and life to be taken over by others. Standing firm in the face of other people wants.

Finding out what really suits YOU and following that. Following and living your own dreams rather than those of others.

Prising away the tentacles of others and their demands.

For helping yourself to not fall into the trap 'I must be seen to be kind and helpful or I am not a good person'.

understanding that you are a worthwhile person and your own needs count.

Notes: Its not at all surprising that I made this essence, in Bach's set I am a Centaury type so Jan's insights totally makes sense.

Jan Rose's insights Centaury types

Rhododendron

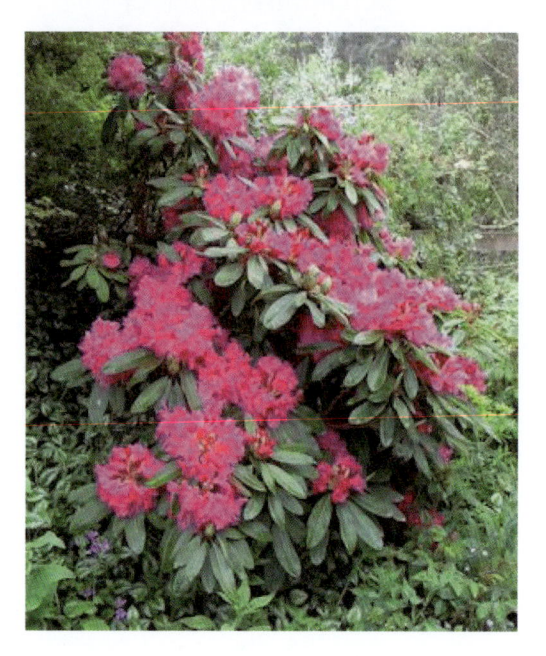

Keywords: boundaries, growth, strength, grounding, vitality, weakness, robust, power, core strength, empowers

Indications: sacrum chakra, solar plexus chakras,
This is an essence which is all about life and vitality. If there is a feeling of disempowerment, it will harness this feeling, helping you to feel back in control and standing in your power.
it can help when we are dealing with over-bearing people, or if we are being overbearing.

Healing Qualities: Good when aging is an issue or people are feeling weakened or disempowered in some way,
Despite circumstantial limitations, we can still be powerful and effective people, enjoying and appreciating our lives and enriching those of others. Strength of spirit.

This essence is about life, vigour and vitality and how the passage of time cannot dim your power and presence (and they may actually be increased by the sum of your life experiences and attitudes).

Notes: When I made this essence I was living with 6 teenagers, so there needed to be clear set boundaries.

Jan Rose's insights
Lively. Invigorating.
Bright green leaves and bright red flowers. Pleasure garden. Elegant fountain. Flower beds. Ladies and gentlemen in Victorian dress promenading around the winding paths. Bandstand with a brass band playing. Some people in seats listening, others on rugs on the grass. A sunny and pleasant scene, keeps fading into watercolours. At the edges are the trees with the vibrant green leaves and bright red flowers. They encircle the scene and are prominent and powerful. Rich, vibrant, alive. The people fade away. The bandstand is now empty and in disrepair. Paths are now straighter and tarmacked. Waste bins. Kids skateboard through. A lot of the flower beds and shrubs have gone, as has the fountain. The trees with their flowers at the periphery have increased and become a thicket encircling the park. Elemental and fairy activity is very strong around them. 19/4/2017 When I made this essence. It is important to note that I was living with 6 teenagers So lots of boundary's needed to be in place. It is a grounding and putting roots down. We were two families who joined together so a busy time of adjustment we were putting our roots down and grounding ourselves.

Rhubarb

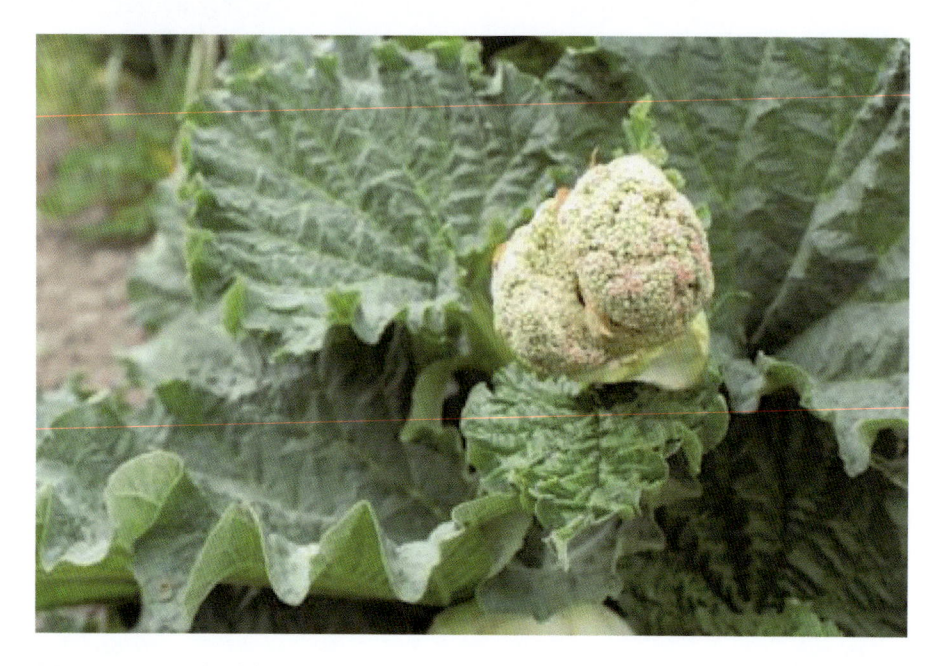

Keywords: timid, anxiety, fear, confidence, flexibility, judgement, resilience, resilience

Indications: solar plexus chakra, sacrum chakra, base chakra
'Can Do Attitude' For when opportunity knocks, but so do the knees. Not sure that you have the confidence to 'Have a go' 'helps us to never give up'.
This essence helps us get back to our core. It helps with the wellbeing of the body.
Rhubarb helps to ground and centre. It takes out the "Ego" identity. And brings us back to into the core of ourselves. Helps to be none judgemental, open hearted.
Brings flexibility to the mind, helping the mind come into alignment with the divine will. Helps with communication between the heart chakra and the mind.

Healing Qualities: This essence was channelled I could feel the strength coming through.

working with it is feels like it brings you back to your core strength.
It helps us deal with the biter sweet in life.
It helps with the Heart and mind communication.

Jan Rose's insights
This essence is for the person who is anxious and timid, they may want to do something but are too scared. 'Instant Confidence in a Bottle'

Rosebay Willowherb

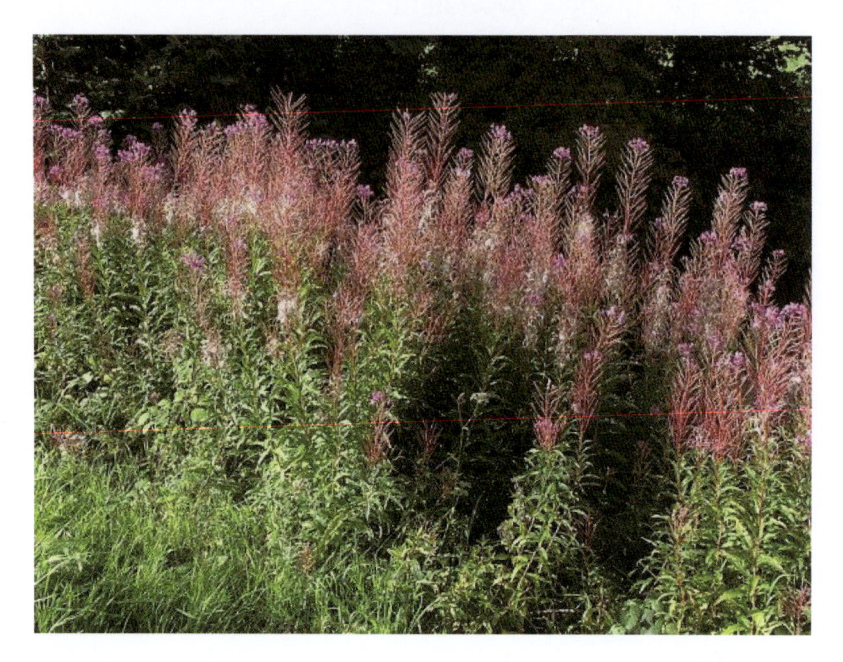

Keywords: grounding, confusion, , disconnection, connection, alert, awareness, confusion, lifts mood, stress, panic, confidence

Indications: Base chakra, Heart, solar plexus, Throat, Crown, connects all the parts of the body.
This a multi faceted essence.
In time of danger or stress , brings your emotions into line so that you are able to make crucial decisions to ensure your safety and survival.
When we are tossed and thrown about by life. Where there is panic, lack of grounding or a situation where important decisions need to made or in life or death scenarios, your emotional balance will be way out, so this essence will bring you back.

Healing Qualities: *Jan Rose's insights*
where people can doubt the innate strength or wisdom of their own body e. g. nervousness before giving birth, elderly people after a fall, 'I won't be able to' 'I'm not strong enough ', 'I won't be well enough'.

Good to use after a therapy session when a client may be content to drift or there is difficulty grounding them and bringing them back to the world, can be put on feet. Useful when a person is too much 'in their own heads' and not fully present.

Notes: I made this essence from a piece of waste land that was really unkept. Despite this, the plant thrives.

Rowan Berry

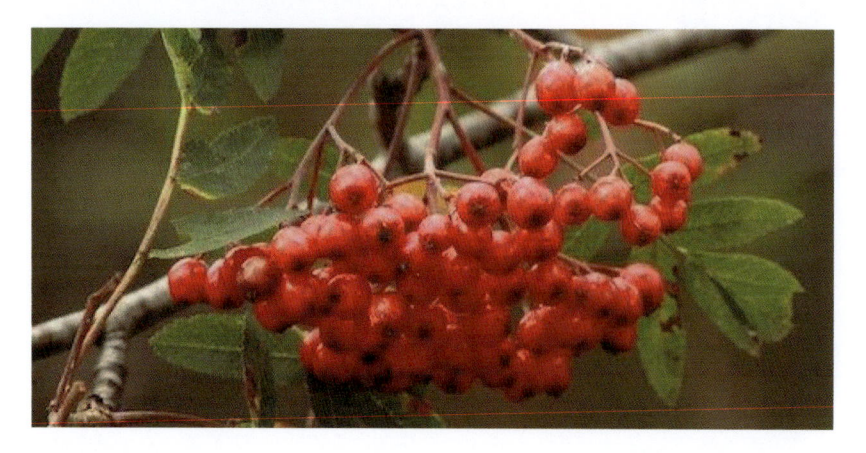

Keywords: all chakra's, overload, head overloaded, protection, grounding, anchor, core strength, power, confidence, diminish

Indications: strengthens the whole chakra system 'All difficulties can be Surmounted' when one feels diminished sapped due to emotional hurt or grief. Gives the strength and will to carry on. 'Lightens the Load'

Healing Qualities: When a person's head is full or overloaded, helps to lighten the load.
It helps to process knowledge gained, and use the knowledge wisely. Is indicated in the base chakra but will strengthen all the chakra's. Good for grounding.

Jan Rose's Insights: Good for when a person, place, or animal is feeling diminished and giving up. Good for the weak or elderly in hospital, helps them to retain their own distinct and individual energies without them becoming compromised or seeping and blending with those of others (alive or in spirit) It is useful for Protection.

Rowan Blossom

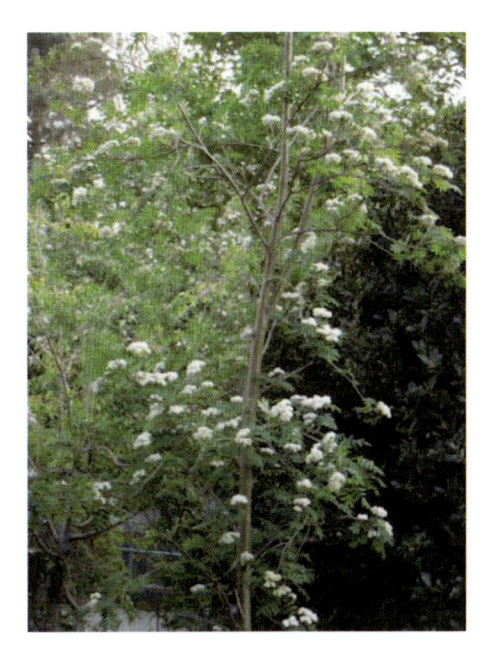

Keywords: protection, responsibility, purifies, peace, reflects

Indications: This essence helps to protect. It reconciles helps us to be at peace with ourselves and others.

Healing Qualities: Rowen flower essence helps us to take responsibility, learning from past experiences, where we have made wrong choices and had to deal with the consequences. Or may be process those choices that we have made but do not realise the consequence.

Scabious

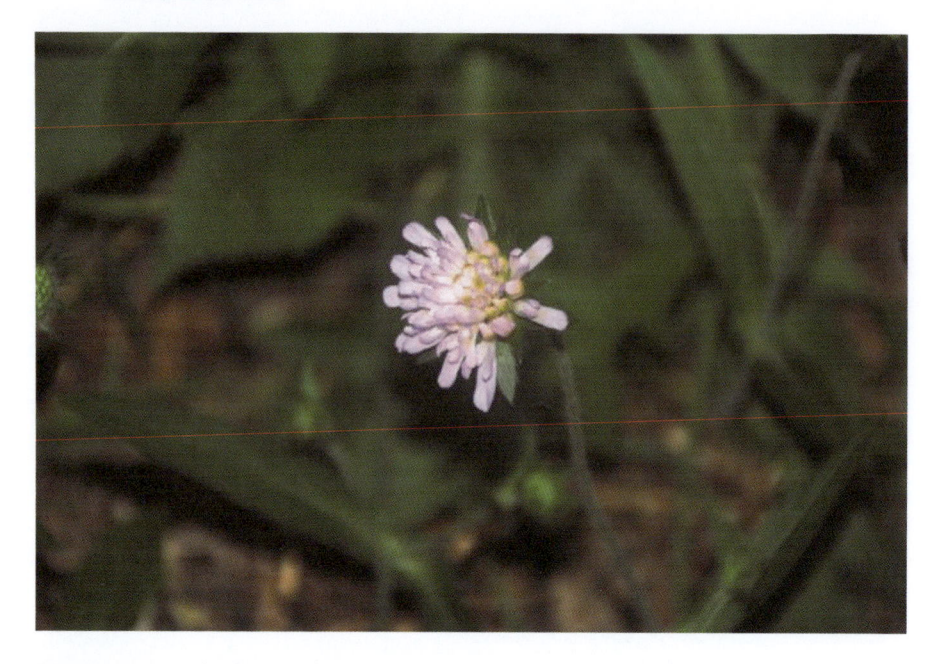

Keywords: clarity, quietens the mind, perseverance, worry, determination, congestion, supportive

Indications: determination to get to where you need to be, quieten the inner chatter.

Healing Qualities: quietens the mind, supports in a gentle way

Self Heal

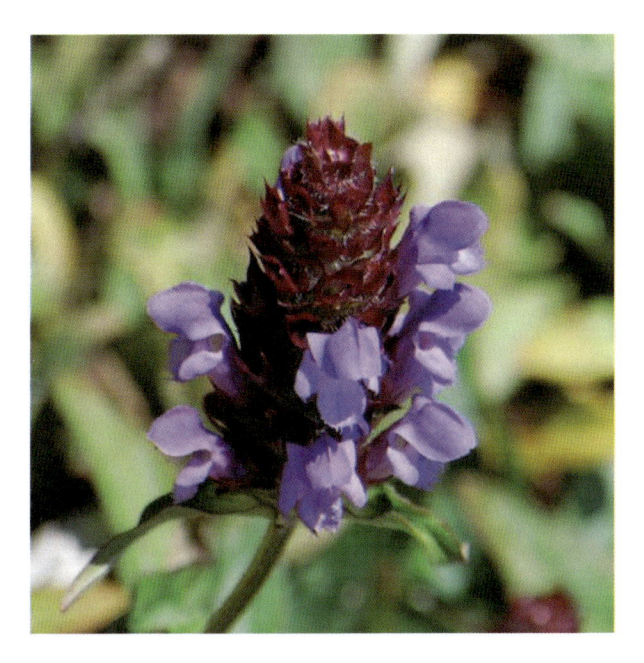

Keywords: clarity, insight, courage, health, understanding, inner strength, balance, gratitude, faith, revives, stuck, gloomy, hope lost, restoration

Indications: Crown, 3rd eye, Heart chakra's. Lines up the Etheric bodies putting you into a state of balance allowing the energy within to flow.
'Faith all will be ok'
Helping people to move when they are stuck, within the restoration process.
Regaining hope that has been lost, restoring faith in yourself and your own inner voice within your own healing process. Living with gratitude for what you have, rather than mourning what you don't. Helping with understanding that there are some things that are just not meant to be, but none the less life is still worthwhile. Things may not be going according to planned but understanding that there is a greater plan is working through us.

Healing Qualities: This essence brings Clarity It brings balance into the thought processes.
It helps us to see other people's points of view.
It gives insight into the self. It gives us the push to help yourself. .
Self-heal helps to listen to our needs of the mind, body and spirit.

Jan Rose's Insights:
Helps to dredge up the reserves of courage and resourcefulness that you would never have known you possessed. When you are dealing with circumstances that are out of ones control.
things may not be going as planned but understanding that there is a greater plan.

Notes: *Jan Rose's insights*
Good in situations where restoration is needed.<

Snow Drop

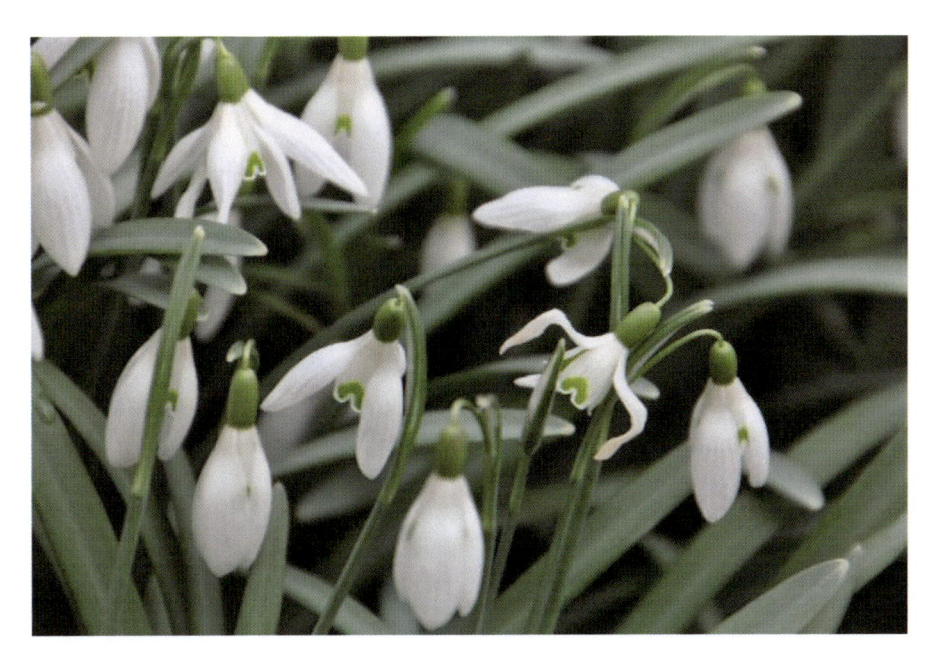

Keywords: strength, grief, heart-break, sadness, conflict, comfort, soothes, joy, rebirth, hope

Indications: Brings strength, for grief and heartbreak, helps to push through sadness and conflict.
It brings comfort and sooths the Heart chakra. Giving hope, it brings new beginnings, filling us with joy.

Healing Qualities: This essence has purity and strength. Snow drop as a plant has a beautiful resilience to it will thrive, it also brings hope, which really come through with the energy of the essence.

Jan Rose's insights
This essence is about grief and heartbreak, even that from long ago. It helps us to take comfort and draw succour from even the smallest of things, aiding our recovery from the sadness's of life. Bringing forth hope rebirth, joy to new beginnings. This essence has purity and strength. Snow drop as a plant has a beautiful resilience to it

will thrive, it also brings hope, which really come through with the energy of the essence.

Notes: When I made this essences I experienced a range of emotions anger, upset, conflict.

Jan Rose's Insights:
Little girl in red Victorian dress bundled up in a thick fur cape with ear muffs and a muffler. Very grave, serious face.
In a graveyard, deep in winter, looking at people gathered around an open grave holding a funeral. She isn't attending this event but is visiting a grave nearby - her mother's. The little girl is silent, numb and desolate, but showing no emotion.
It is bitterly, freezing cold. She is comforted by the warmth of her cape and the ear muffs and muffler. Their softness and warmth reminds her of her new kitten waiting at home. The thought gives her comfort and something to look forward to on this bleak day.

Sycamore

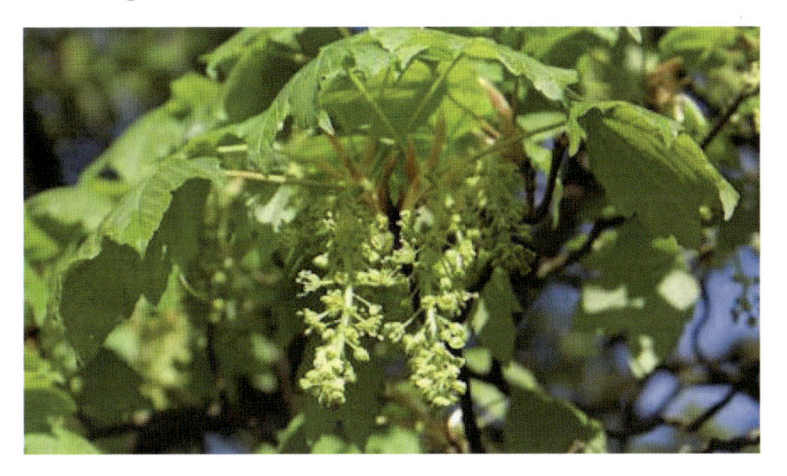

Keywords: sweetness, nurturing, self, mother hen, emotional blockages, release, soothes, fear, emotions

Indications: 3rd eye chakra, throat chakra, heart chakra, Solar Plexus chakra.
'Bringing the sweetness back in. Healing old hurts, of the heart chakra gently clears emotional blockages, releasing from emotional baggage.

Healing Qualities: Where there has been deep hurt in the past it helps to releases those hurts and bring the sweetness back in. sooths on a deep level.

Jan Rose's insights Useful too for those who will not allow themselves to be nurtured or mothered (maybe because of bad experiences in the past) but who instead 'Mother Hen' everyone else. Helps them to accept help for themselves and to drop the reins and only offer help to others if they have been asked to, rather than try to help and then be hurt when people rebuff them. To accept nurturing for the self; for mother hen type; for mothering, nurturing. Soothing fears and emotions Gently clearing emotional blockages. Releasing. Settling fears and emotions. Healing.
Good all round essence that could form the basis for many

combinations or dosage bottles. Could be applied directly to the Solar Plexus or the corresponding point on the feet.

Notes: Uncomfortable turbulent feeling in stomach. Churned up. Can feel hands smoothing the stomach and Solar Plexus - they begin in the middle and then pull the energy outwards. Clearing.
One hand on the stomach, the other on the Solar Plexus. Steadying and stabilising it. One hand on the front of the solar Plexus, the other on the back. Holding it there. Warmth.

Torbay Palm

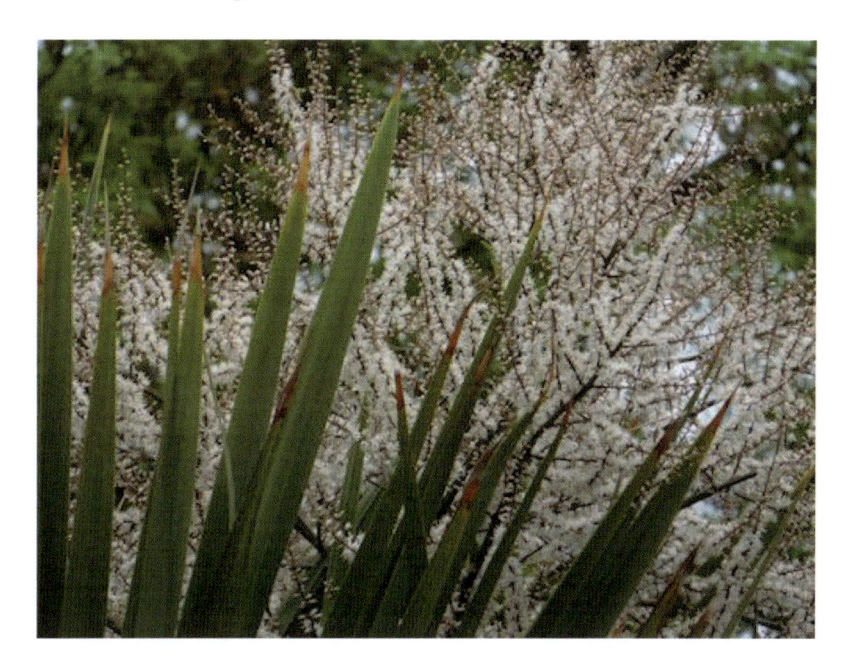

Keywords: regeneration, adaptability, cheerfulness, fulfilment, agitation, emotion blockages, homesick, displaced, ancestral, challenges, rawness, adoption, roots, anchor

Indications: 3rd eye, throat chakra, heart chakra, solar plexus, sacrum chakra, root chakra,
This is an essence that will help regenerate after facing challenges that have taken us to the brink of our inner and outer reserves.

Helps you fit in and feel at home wherever you are.
Lightness of being. Enjoyment of life and a sense of contentment whoever you are whatever you are doing.

Healing Qualities: Torbay palm is like a beacon of light, helping to follow our own light showing the way.
'Like a phoenix rising up out of the ashes' in many ways sums this amazing essence up. Regeneration - this is one of the first plants to

grow after fire, and it can produce a million seeds on one flower head.

Notes: *Jan Rose's insights*
Helps you to put down roots and thriving wherever you are and what ever circumstances.

For those who are displaced or with out roots i.e. immigrants, homeless, in insecure accommodation.
For those who feel they do not fit in. Pining to be elsewhere or someone else, feeling that who they actually are is not right or not good enough. Not knowing who you are.
For those torn between two or more cultures, feeling that they do not fit in or belong completely to either world. Making peace with this and celebrating their uniqueness.

where there has been an irreversible and permanent life change, learning to live and make the best possible life within that framework.

Rustling and sounds of wind around the head.

Rafe Nauen's insights: In 2008 after a hard winter the Torbay Palm was dead. I took down the trunk, and left the rotting roots behind - partly to enable other plants to remain undisturbed, but also because I'm a lazy gardener. A full two years went by with no change. Within four years, the Torbay Palm was back to full glory, and flowering - very much a phoenix from the ashes

Turkish-Filbert

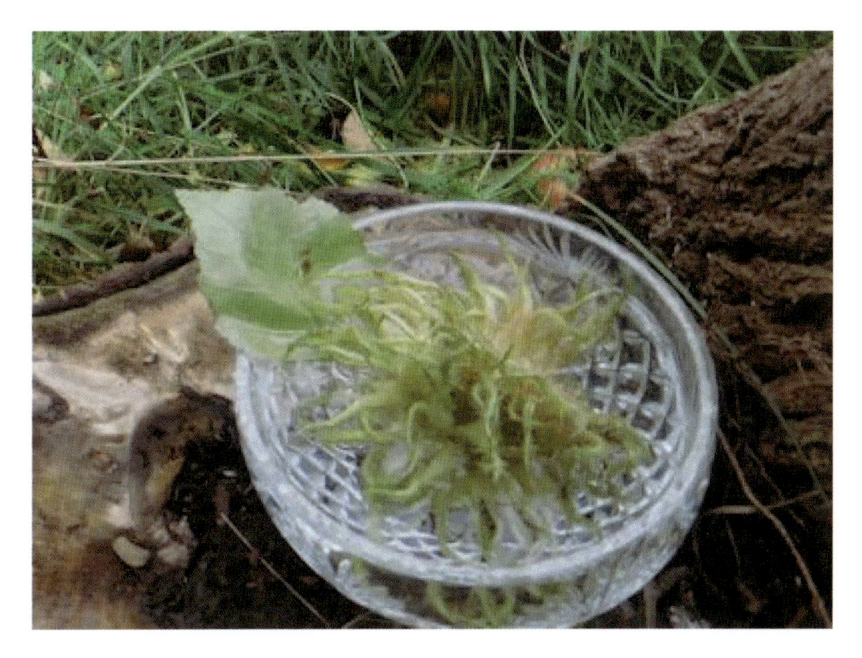

Keywords: child-like, wonder, delight, veil lifter, nourishment, protection, supportive, uplifts,

Indications: Throat chakra, an essence that is beneficial , helps one feel protected, nourished, supported.

Healing Qualities: I want for nothing, thus I can give everything. It helps one feel protected, nourished supported enough so one can give of oneself, even in difficult and challenging times. The energy from this essence uplifts, brings a natural protection.

I was so bolled over with the seed I had never seen, this before so it was a beautiful new experience.

Notes: it is part of the Hazel-Nut family.

Viburnum Burkwoodii

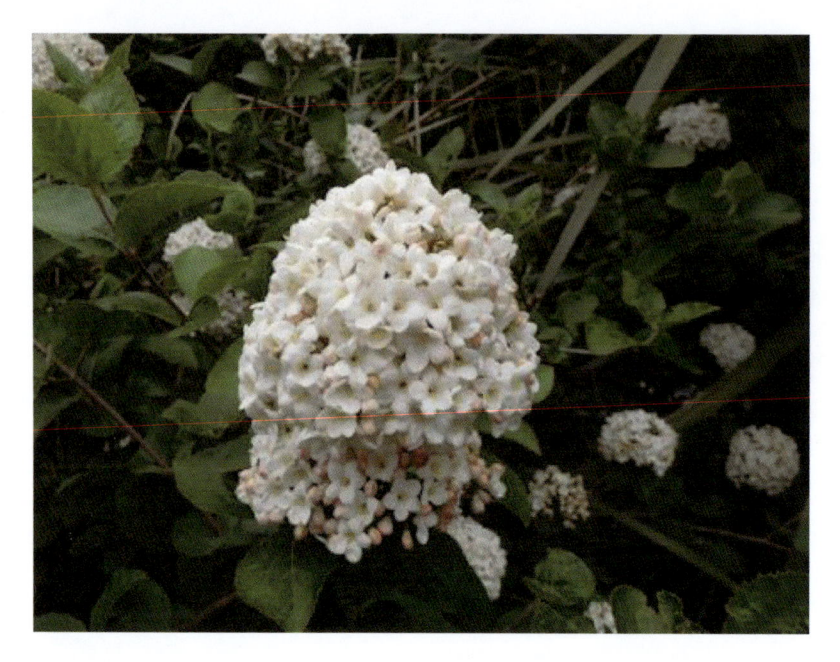

Keywords: support, reassure, vulnerable, unhappy, identity, direction, hidden knowledge, Akashic records, dreams, , meditations, grounds

Indications: This reassuring essence will help with feelings of vulnerability, it will help establish identity and direction
This will help to access and down load information

Healing Qualities: *Jan Rose's insights*
This essence supports and reassures, when there is a feeling of vulnerability.
information that is needed will come to you through dreams, meditation, journeying or in your thinking. it increases receptivity so that spirit can get through to you. It will enable you to stay grounded and retain the information, using it to your advantage.
would combine well with Laurel.

Notes: This heavy scented flower has an ethereal quality about it. Would combine well with Laurel.

White Dog Rose

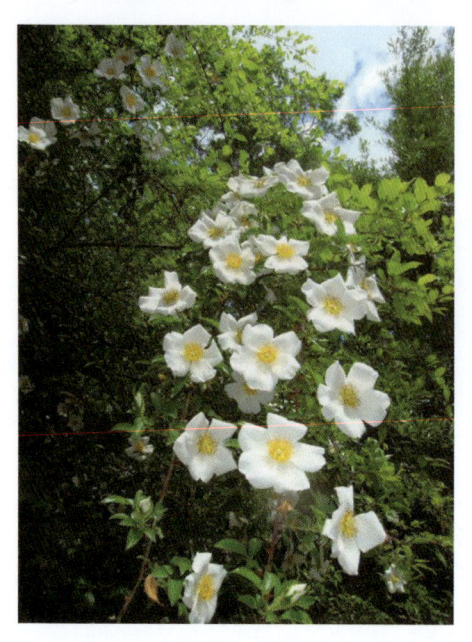

Keywords: simplicity, complicated

Indications: Dog rose is all about simplicity. Getting back to basics. Reminding us who we are.

Healing Qualities: The quality this brings as an essence, is that when life becomes too complicated than it will help us simplify, taking us back to basics so things feel far simpler. Nothing has changed only the way we deal with life.

White Hawthorn

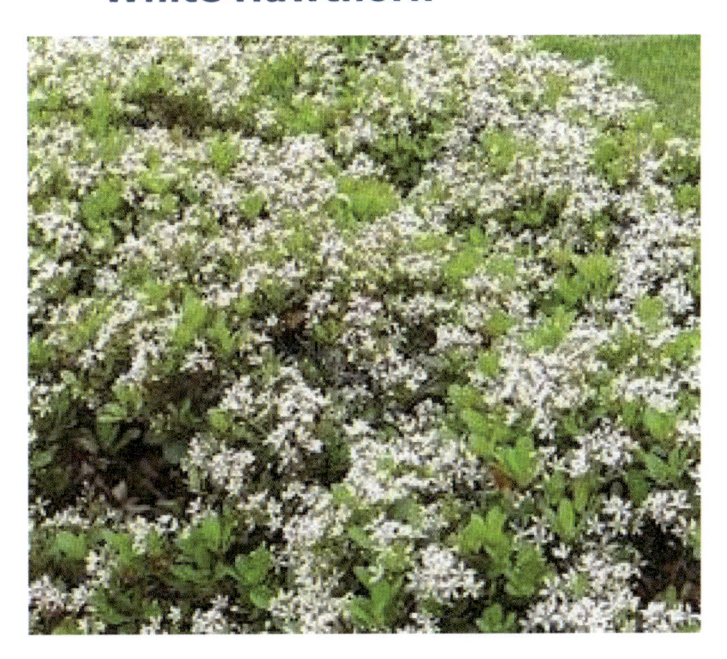

Keywords: light, hope, resets, settles, transitions, new beginnings, strength, patience, quiet strength, steadfastness, tenacity, clarity, discernment, judgement, decision, impartial, remote viewing, divorce

Indications: Bringing the light back in. It resets after major life events. Divorce, house move. etc.
it gives an overview of situations helping to remain impartial

Healing Qualities: It helps to settle and reassure during new beginnings and transitions, giving us the tools to move forward. Bringing with it clarity to see clearly. So we can accurately pinpoint reason's and causes for situations and how to fix them.

Notes: Hawks eye view of entire landscape and situation.
brings clarity.

White Lilac

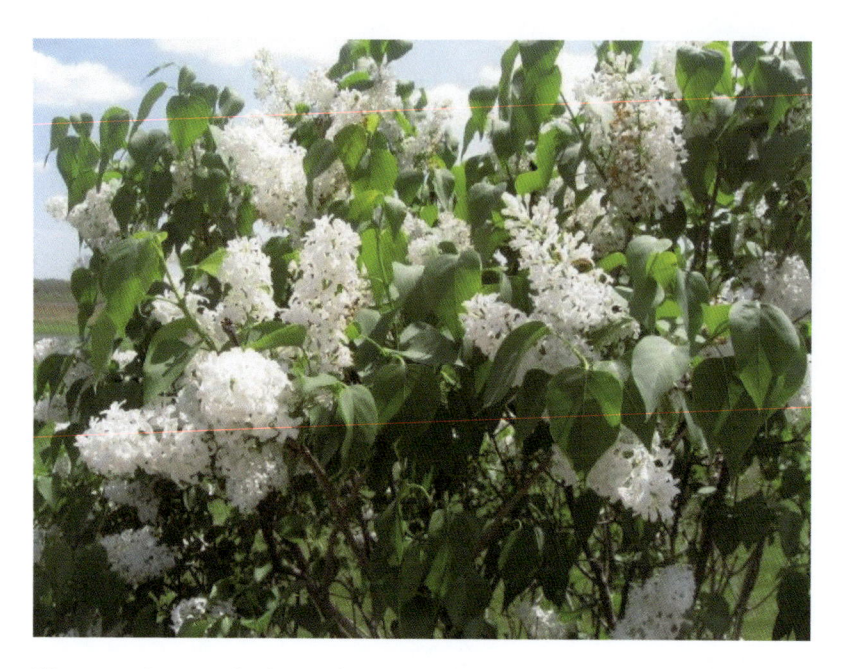

Keywords: confusion, chaos, clears, cleanses, negativity, protection, purity,

Indications: crown chakra, heart chakra, sacrum chakra,
Helps us not get caught up in negativity of material world. For protection and clearing

Healing Qualities: This essence will protect when we are surrounded by chaos. There is massive protection with this essence protecting us from chaos. Also on a psychic level it will protect us from other peoples ill-wishes keeping us clear protecting our energy field.
White Lilac shows us the truth, beauty and perfection that is always around us and available, even throughout (or especially!) our earthly trials and tests. It helps us to see the bigger spiritual picture and avoid being caught up in the negativity of the material world.
Even when life is an uphill struggle and you feel beset on all sides, look up to the Heavens and absorb what is real and true.

This essence is about connection to the Creator and the Cosmos. When this link is strong, only truth and purity can abide.

Notes: When Lilac came to my notice, it had split away from the main trunk. After making the essences I began to realise that it was an essence for protection. At the time I was being subjected to psychic attack. White lilac was really an effective protector. This was backed up by Jan's information which followed latter making total sense after what I had encountered.

Jan Roses insights
Cold in palm. Heart chakra. Brightness of the emerging dawn. I keep gazing at this vast and timeless beauty and realise that the night sky is giving way to the
See a windswept darkening hillside. Moorland. Ruined building on brow.
Walking up a winding path to the top. Wind whistling and howling around me, light fading. The path peters out as I reach the top. Plateau. Wind still whistling shrilly but now intermingled with faint voices too.
Stand looking at the ruin. The wind shrieks by, the discarnates call as they whip past. So many of them.
The discarnates try to intimidate me by whistling past, very close, calling. They move around in a figure of 8, with me at the centre. Within this centre I am totally safe.
I allow them to do their worst. I look up at the inky black sky peppered with bright stars. The calm night sky, the purity of the Heavens, the beauty of the eternal Cosmos - all help to put the antics of these entities into their proper perspective. No fear or turmoil can enter such perfection.
See a windswept darkening hillside. Moorland. Ruined building on brow. Walking up a winding path to the top. Wind whistling and howling around me, light fading. The path peters out as I reach the top. Plateau. Wind still whistling shrilly but now intermingled with faint voices too.
Stand looking at the ruin. The wind shrieks by, the discarnates call as they whip past. So many of them.
I feel no fear. I simply stand and observe, knowing that I am safe and

protected.

The discarnates try to intimidate me by whistling past, very close, calling. They move around in a figure of 8, with me at the centre. Within this centre I am totally safe.

I allow them to do their worst. I look up at the inky black sky peppered with bright stars. The calm night sky, the purity of the Heavens, the beauty of the eternal Cosmos - all help to put the antics of these entities into their proper perspective. No fear or turmoil can enter such perfection.

The wind drops, the discarnates howl their last. All is still and right with the world. I feel no fear. I simply stand and observe, knowing that I am safe and protected.

White Rambling Rose

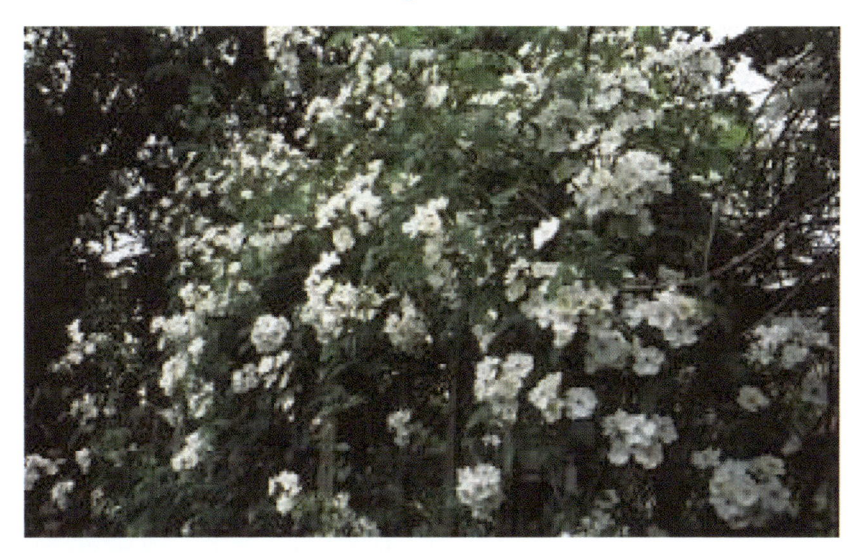

Keywords: cushions, flexibility, soothing, fragile, emotional rawness, vulnerable

Indications: 3rd Eye chakra, heart chakra.
Like sitting on a cloud or cushion, for people who are fragile and emotionally raw. Suitable for vulnerable people and animals.

Healing Qualities: Soothing and balancing, going to wherever it is needed.
Bringing back into alignment.
Earthing and flexibility.
Very supportive of any healing treatments; would be lovely as a spray in a therapy room. A good base for a lot of dosage bottles, especially where clients are fragile and emotions are raw. Good to put on hands and/or around a space when working with animal. Its soothing gentle action will settle vulnerable clients. Connecting. Returning to wholeness.

Notes: *Jan Rose's experiences*
Becoming very aware of Head midway between 3rd Eye and Crown. Ears. Temples. Soles of feet.

Cooling. Calming. Cushioning.
Base chakra. Soles of feet.

White Sage

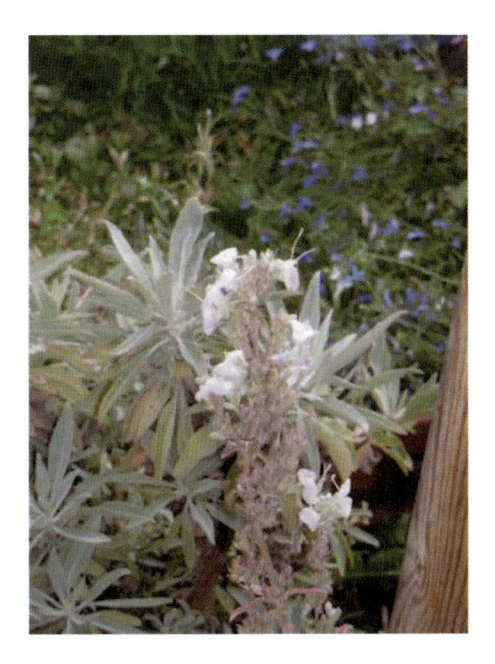

Keywords: cleanse, purifies, aura

Indications: It is an excellent essence as it clears out on so many levels. Cleansing the Aura, the emotional field and the mind. Clears heavy negative thoughts and feelings.

Healing Qualities: This essence is for cleansing and clearing out. It has the wisdom to go where it needs to go. It clears dark dense energies, and lifts the energy that this energy creates. It puts back a lightness into your whole being.
White sage has the wisdom to helps us reconnect with what we have been cut off from. Can be added to baths and to sprays

Notes: I grew this fabulous plant from seed and when it came into flower I just knew it was a gift. So The tiny very pale lilac flowers really made the most beautiful essence. So thank you to the wisdom of the sage.

White Spirea

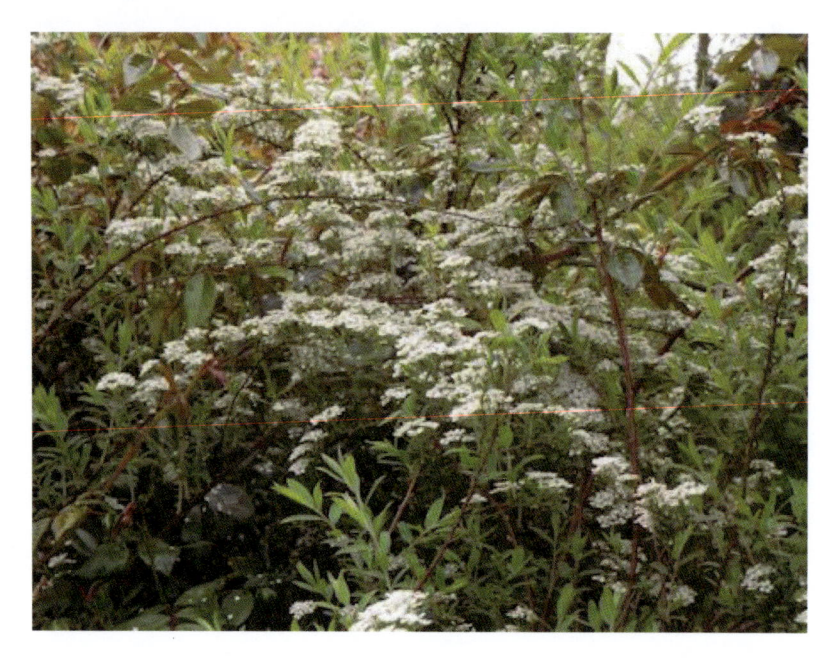

Keywords: balances chakras, focus, realigns, higher perspective,

Indications: crown, 3rd eye, throat chakra, solar plexus,
This essence helps with focus. It also realigns. Listening to what is and isn't being said. Seeing what is really there and what isn't being obviously shown. Seeing through illusion and 'glamour'.

Healing Qualities: This essence know what it is about it, it focuses its energy bringing balance to the Chakras. One of its main functions is to realign.

Jan Rose's insights
Brings in awareness on all levels. Utilising all senses to their fullest potential and abilities.
Becoming a fully awake and aware human being.
It helps open you up to spirit and All-That-Is. Clear contact and communication. Becoming a clear pure channel.

Good for therapists, mediums, spiritual workers and those who are just setting out on this path: clears the airwaves to receive, use and pass on information. For becoming fully awakened and aware. Higher perspective. Acute awareness of your surroundings and all that is occurring within them.

Notes: *Jan Rose's insights*
Vortex whirling out from it, transmitting, seeking out, trying to make contact. Could work with Cornflower

Wild Garlic

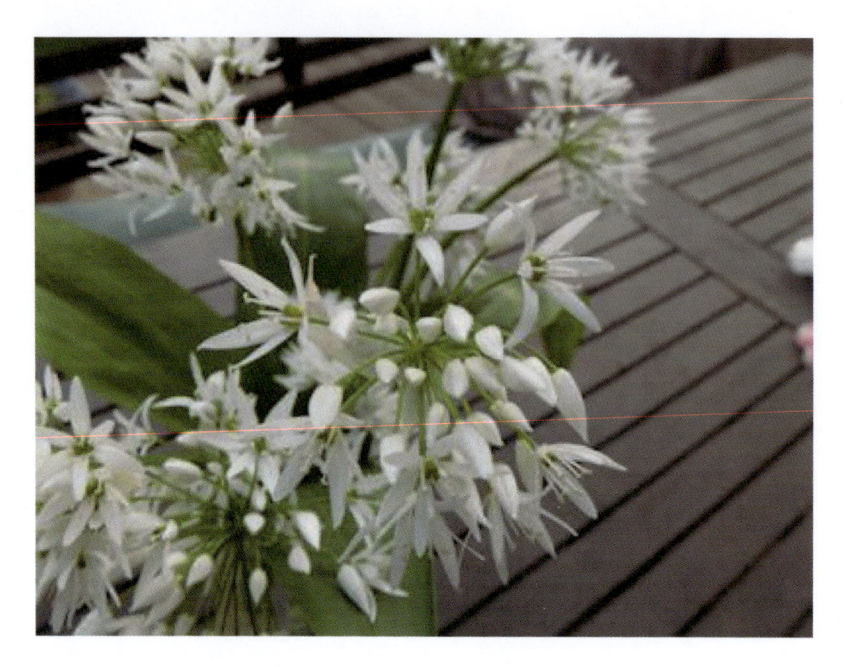

Keywords: protection, uplifts, safe, clears, cleanses,

Indications: This essences, protects, and uplifts. Holding a space safely and effectively so that new healthy growth may emerge.

Healing Qualities: *Jan Rose's insights*
we can call in the collective spirit of Wild Garlic in its entirety. It cleanses clears, uplifts, and brings strength. For people, animals and places. It will be good to use in therapy or meeting rooms, schools or hospitals. It is also really effective for places, people and animals which have been defiled and disrespected.

Notes: The dell I made this in had a clear energy. The place felt magical and very easy.

Willow

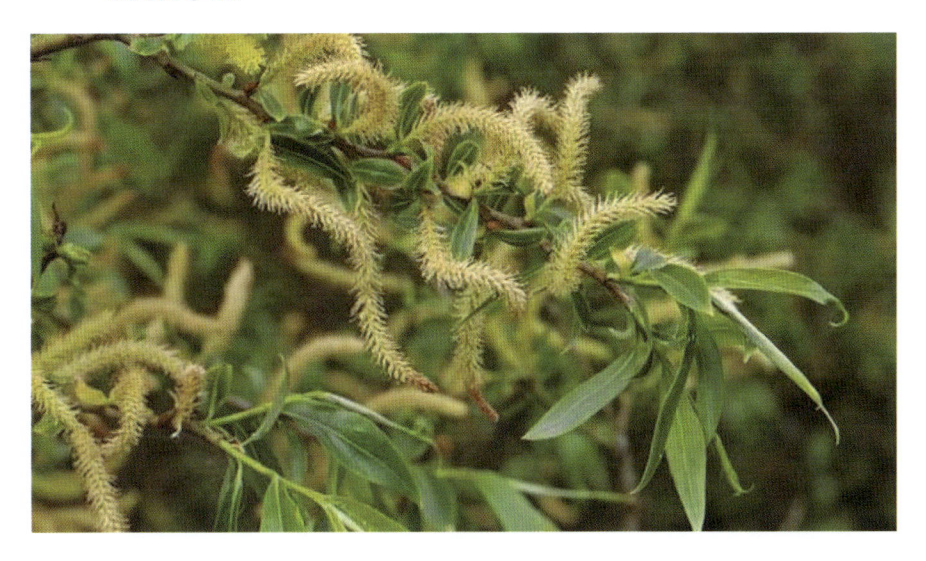

Keywords: clarity, gateway, flexibility, wisdom, overwhelmed,

Indications: useful for therapists, and clients when swamped.

Healing Qualities: swamped by our emotions, feelings of emotional drowning helps one feel separate from the mental and emotional craziness. This essence helps find peace and not get pulled into the turmoil. Gives us greater understanding.

Helen Ward observations This is a gift from spirit, giving us clarity and depth in our perception of what are our affairs and what are others. Useful for therapists it will help with explanation about what may have been absorbed from the energy that surrounds them and this essence helps to disconnect, from the draining overwhelming energies

Wisteria

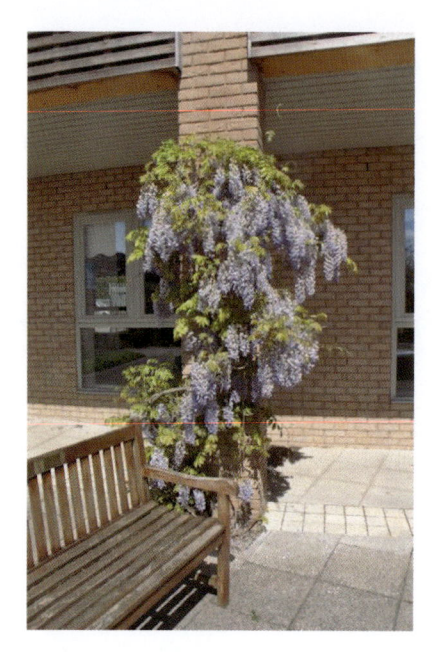

Keywords: grief, deep sadness, embedded, release, rawness, peace

Indications: If you are feeling raw or have experienced deep embedded grief this essence will help settle down the emotions.

Healing Qualities: This essence is all about deep grief leaving you feeling raw. It helps release deeply embedded trapped emotions that we are holding.
As I made the essence I became very emotional. I started to cry. But then there came a huge sense of peace.

Notes: This essence came from a conversation with Andrew Tresider. He said I needed to make an essence out of Wisteria. I didn't know where I was going to find this flower but left it and trusted it to the universe. As I went to vote on the Thursday morning. There it was in full bloom. It made me smile!
I went back the following day. The morning I made it was the day after the general election. In the church next door a funeral was

taking place for a young man had who had committed suicide. It was a huge affair.

This essence seems to bring a sense of emotional peace through and after grief.

When I came home I took the essence and started to cry deep sobs, as quickly as that well of emotion came it then lifted and a sense of peace returned.

Yellow-Poppy

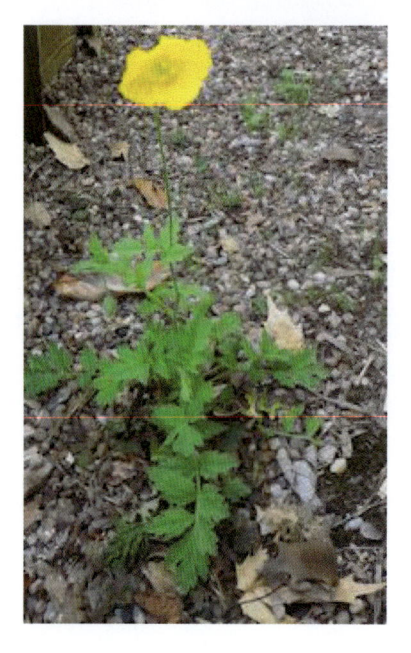

Keywords: Strength, Fragile, vulnerable

Indications: when we feel vulnerable, fragile and ungrounded.

Healing Qualities: These beautiful yellow flowers appear fragile, but their roots go deep and are incredibly strong. Yellow poppy helps us discover just how strong we are. In times when we feel vulnerable and fragile will help to strengthen and ground.

Essences made at the Field Ilkeston

Angelica seed

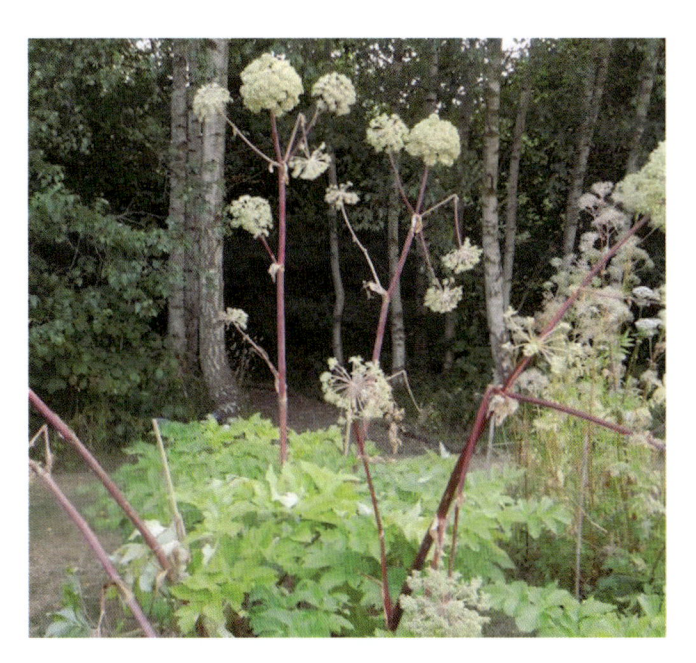

Keywords: chakras, third eye, solar plexus, Clarity, decisive, reflect, transitions, strength, healing, inner guidance, inner self, protection, psychic connections. networker

Indications: Pineal, Crown, 3rd eye. During transitional times this essence will give space to be able to reflect without being emotional. Helps put you back in touch with your inner self, connecting you with your inner guidance. Use for Spiritual Support and Protection. Helps with psychic connections. A great net worker.

Healing Qualities: Helps to create space within to reflect on life's experiences, which will bring about realisations and healing of the past putting you where you need to be. Angelica Seed has lots of strength, which in turn passes onto the recipient supporting giving strength. This helps get you back in touch with your inner guidance it may help with end of life transitions

Notes: Really out of sorts after making Echinacea. This had been left over night. Remained really out of sorts whilst this essence was being birthed. Forgot a client. Lots of reflection took place, remembered my fathers violence. Remembered the plants at the garden reflected and gave thanks. It was Left overnight until the following day. When I went to collect this essence, I sat listening to radio 2 folk hour. Pluto back after being retrograde. Pineal, pituitary

Belladonna

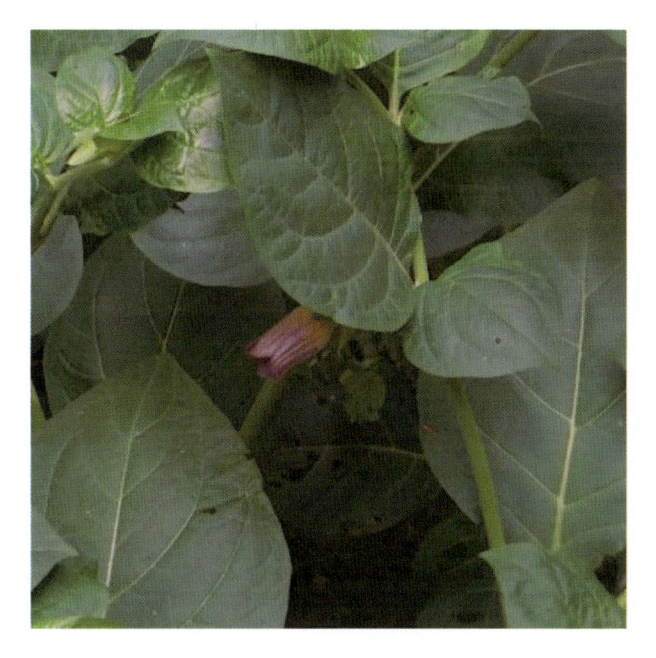

Keywords: self esteem, negative body-image, anorexia, distorted view, clarity

Indications: For those who have a distorted view of themselves, body image, no self value.
it can also help to connect with the elementals
Can help access to different realms, Fairy's and magical worlds

Healing Qualities: This can help with poor body image, a distorted view may have anorexia, or Issues with how one looks. Some where along the line there has been a negative frequency that has taken hold which has become a vibrational knot of twisted energy. Belladonna, helps cut through illusion, the contrast between dark and light brings clarity.
Where there is a distorted opinion on situations Belladonna helps give a clearer understanding of the truth at the heart of the matter.

Notes: Belladonna, *deadly nightshade* - beautiful woman in Italian. Used in Renaissance times to dilate pupils. It was made into eyedrops from the berries. Not used in the present day because of its high toxicity.
it is used in medicines today as a muscular relaxant.

Black Cohosh

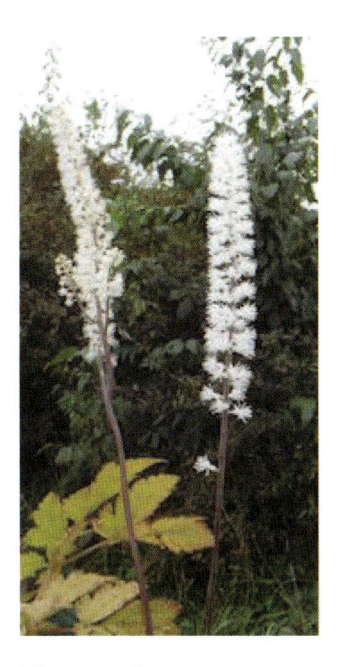

Keywords: courage, transformation, realignment, balance, cleansing, energises, puberty, pregnancy, birth, motherhood, menopause, wise woman, crone, letting go, loss, peace, fear, attachments, abuse

Indications: Black Cohosh for powerful transformation. In child birth to help with the process of letting go. Useful support for major life changes, stepping into those changes, particularly for woman e.g. puberty, pregnancy, birth, menopause and beyond into the wise woman and crone stages of being a woman.

Healing Qualities: This essence was birthed on the Autumn equinox in 2019, which is about bringing things back into balance. Black Cohosh works with all the chakras. Works with the communication pathways of the body. Harnessing the wisdoms within. When we are walking right on the edge, Black cohosh gives the courage to let go. It can help to heal past abuse issues that have penetrated deep within. Helps deal with loss and our shadow side, transforming those into the positive.

Notes: Autumn Equinox 2019. all about bringing in the balance.

Black-Eyed-Susan (Rudbeckia)

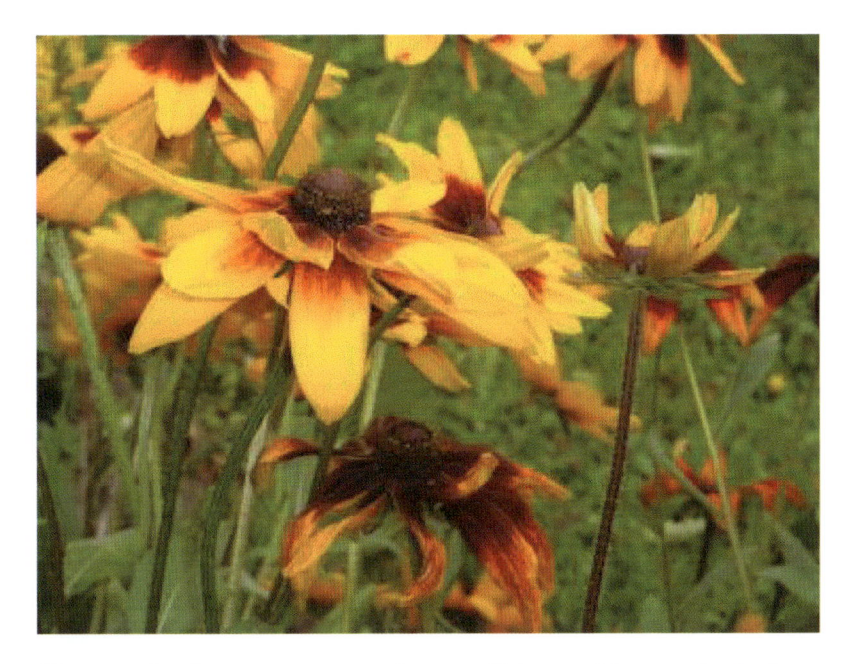

Keywords: burn out, strength, true Grit, positive outlook, inner resources

Indications: Black eyed Susan gives a positive outlook, stopping you in your tracks.

Healing Qualities: The song that came to mind was "slow down you move too fast" Simon and Garfunkel.

Helen Wards insights, Saw an Iron fist in her middle, representing the strength this essence brings with it. It helps to smash what is no longer needed, helping to beat the odds, even when things seem impossible. It will help to initiate and apply more positive viewpoints, so that the essence can then draw on the more useful resources' within. True strength need good foundation, and this essence will help one start building anew.

Notes: this essence certainly tried to rush me I woke really early when it was still dark. But wasn't happy about walking in the field in the Dark. Going back to sleep I asked to be woken early at first light, I woke at 6 am. Two indications. Being rushed and stopping in my tracks.

Blackthorn

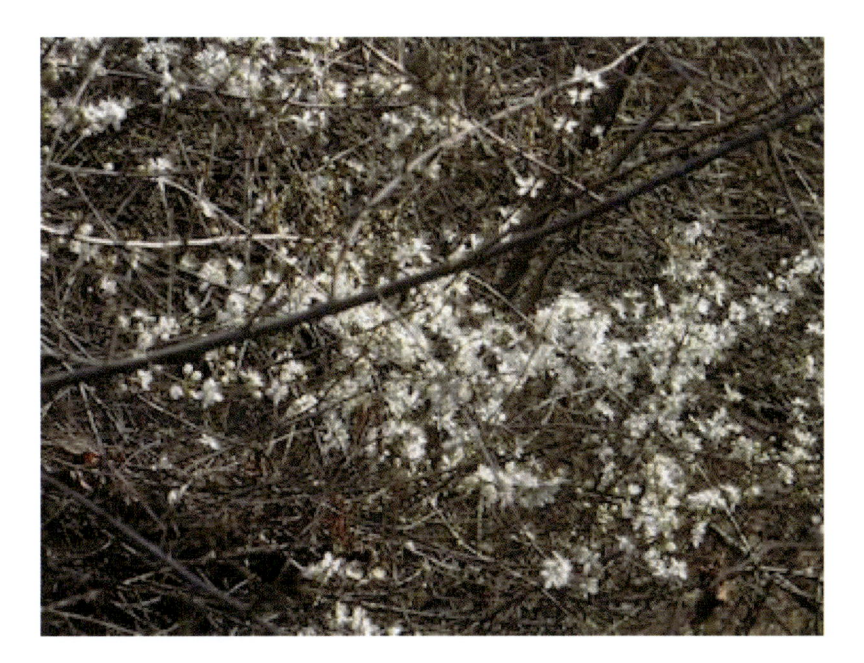

Keywords: balances, calms, clears, supportive, stabilises, protective, purifies, renews, hope, joy, burdened, fatigue, toxic, weary, despair, fester,

Indications: "Bridge over Troubled Waters" sums up this essence. Useful when we are burdened by life, fatigued and weary, feels like no support. No hope or joy. When things are festering in our thoughts it will help to clear the head.

Healing Qualities: "Bridge over troubled waters" was the song that came to mind when this essence was birthed. Stabilises the emotions, bringing hope, joy, and balance. Purifies the negative, Clears out the clutter of old wounds that are toxic and festering, that will destroy. It will also help to protect from those influences when we are tired and feel dragged down by life this puts us into a venerable state.

Notes: As I was gearing up to this essence being made. I became very weary feeling burdened.

Boneset-Eupatorium-Perfoliatum

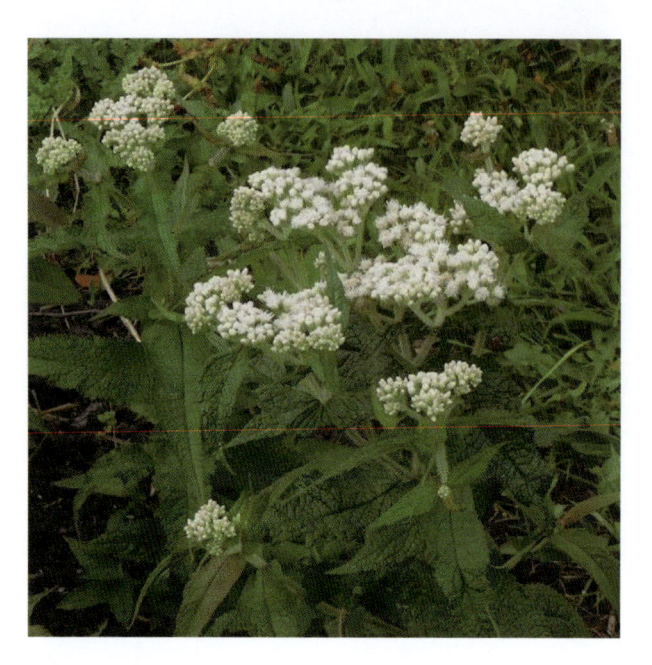

Keywords: exhaustion, depleted, resets, release, reorientates, meridians, surrendering, unblocks,

Indications: meridians, zero balances,

Healing Qualities: letting go , surrendering to the process. Slow but powerful essence.
I was really out of kilter when this essence was being created, dealing with anger issues of things that life had dealt me. When the essence had been created it was like the curtain lifted, this has been my experience on so many occasions. It was like I was taken into a complete state of balance.

Notes: The night before this essence was birthed I was beyond exhausted. The day I went to co-create this essence my cameras battery was exhausted. Also my bones in my legs deeply ached, a sore throat which suddenly came on.
Helen Ward's insights, ' let go and sink into a deeper peacefulness',

as 'doing' is not possible right now. 'Although, I seem to be quite still, my 'inner body' is moving around, re-orienting it's basic energies- meridians shifting, flows unblocking'

Boneset is part of the Aster family nothing to do with comfrey. As a herb it was used by the Native Americans to treat fever, it has Anti Viral properties, they used it to treat 'Break Bone fever' Dengue Fever, the pain in the bones was so intense that they thought their bones would break.

Borage

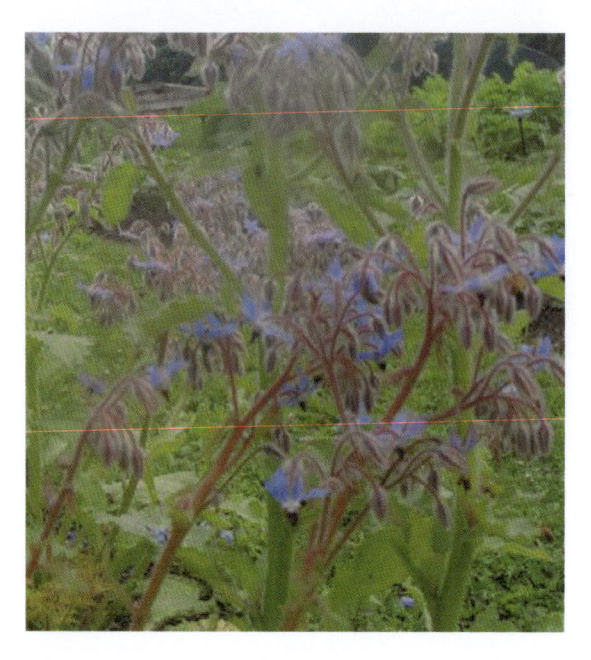

Keywords: fear, grief, loneliness, Identification, nurturing. Community

Indications: surrounded by nurturing experiences.

Healing Qualities: when I arrived at the field to co-create this essence there were some children taking part in a Forestry school. I was also going to see my own Grand children, after which I went home and spent the day in the garden. All of these experiences to me spoke of nurturing a coming together.

Helen wards insights 'This essences definitely links into loneliness, and not having the right place or position in life, not having the relating component as you'd like it. This is all about identification, for when the person is having trouble.

Notes: calm cloudy day, Borage is a beautiful blue, 5 petaled star shaped flower. Some of the flowers are almost pink, the flowers come in clusters. Lots of bees around they love Borage. The gesture of the flowers face down, some are open some are closed. The stems lots of course fine hairs, the leave have lots of veins. There are no flowers for the first foot. The atmosphere is really peaceful. Later when I went to pick the essence up 3 flowers had fallen into the water.

As a woman's herb it is called Star Flower, can be used for PMS .

Calendula

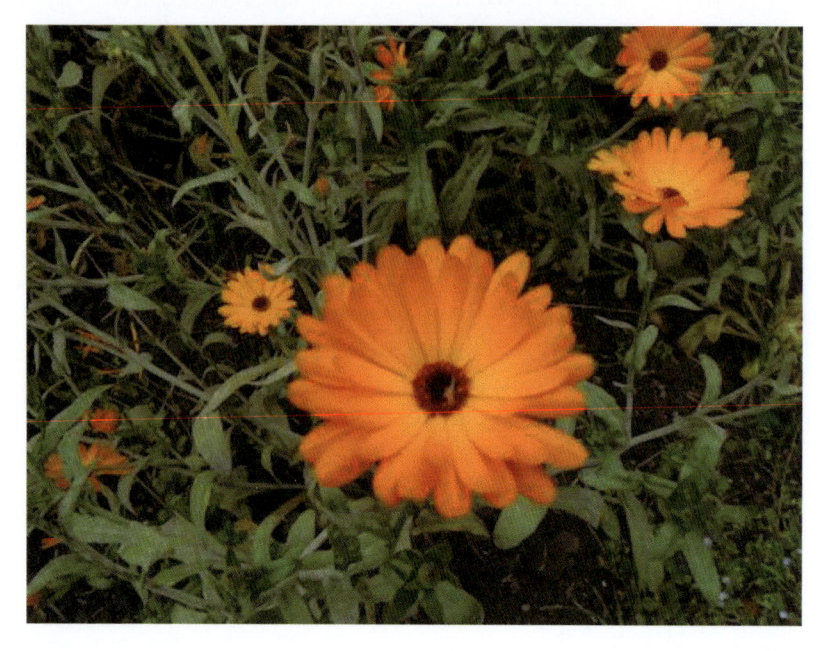

Keywords: throat, mouth, deep sadness, depression, melancholia, chaos, orders sunshine, laughter, happiness, vitality, sunshine lift

Indications: Heart Centre. Excellent for those who need to let some sunshine into their lives.
Use as a room spray to prime a place ahead of a party or gathering. Helps to engender good will and an enjoyment of company.

Healing Qualities: 'you are my sunshine' This Sunshine essence, brings a warmth and vitality, but not excessive or full-on.
It gives you a feeling of being lighter and like smiling. Content and wanting to spread that feeling to others.

Helps with feelings of deep sadness that are dragging into a place of misery bringing a lightness to the heart, helping to open the Heart, of the receptivity to love, laughter, happiness, friendship and all the good things in life.

Brings lightness, inner and outer smiling. Content and wanting to spread that feeling to others.

Good for priming place ahead of a party or gathering, will help to engender goodwill and an enjoyment of company.
Excellent for those who need to let sunshine into their lives.

Notes: *Jan Rose's Insights: Heart centre, seeing golden petals folding and unfolding. Golden glow around the heart, moving outwards to fill the whole body and beyond.*
Very attractive to 'little people, especially if they are feeling disgruntled with people and their behaviour; makes them feel happier and less resentful
Very attractive to the 'Little people', especially if they are feeling a bit disgruntled with people and their behaviour; makes them feel happier and less resentful.

Opening the heart. Receptivity to love, laughter, happiness, friendship and all the really good things in life.

Chamomile

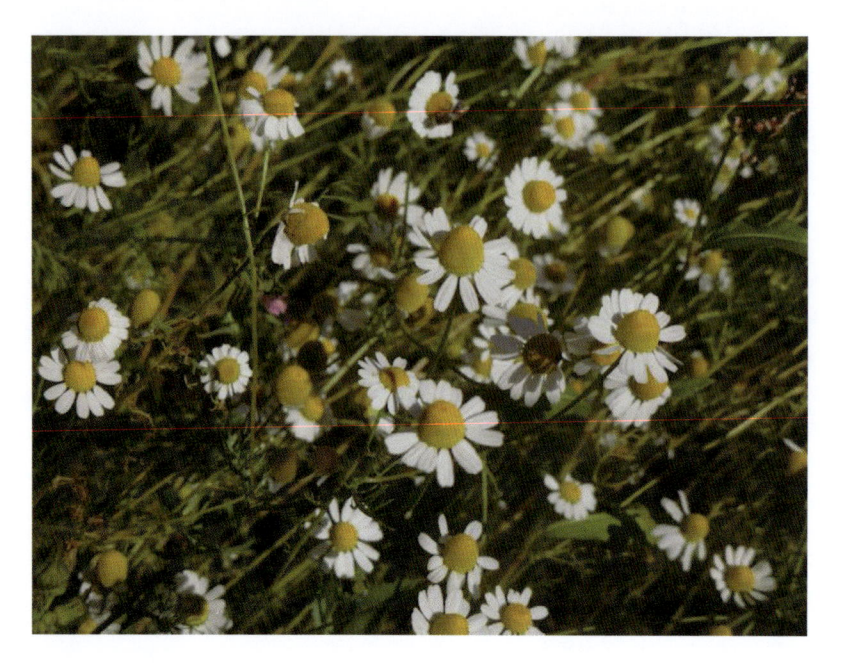

Keywords: slumber, sleep, letting-go, relax, focus, anger, conflict, irritation, lightens mood, stress, chillax

Indications: Soothes anger, conflict and irritation. Helps with tensions and emotional unease. It helps stop the accumulating effects that build up through the day. Helps you to be more settled at night.

Healing Qualities: helps to deal with the stress and strains that build up through the day. This in turn helps with being more settled at night and generally more relaxed in ones manner.

Chicory

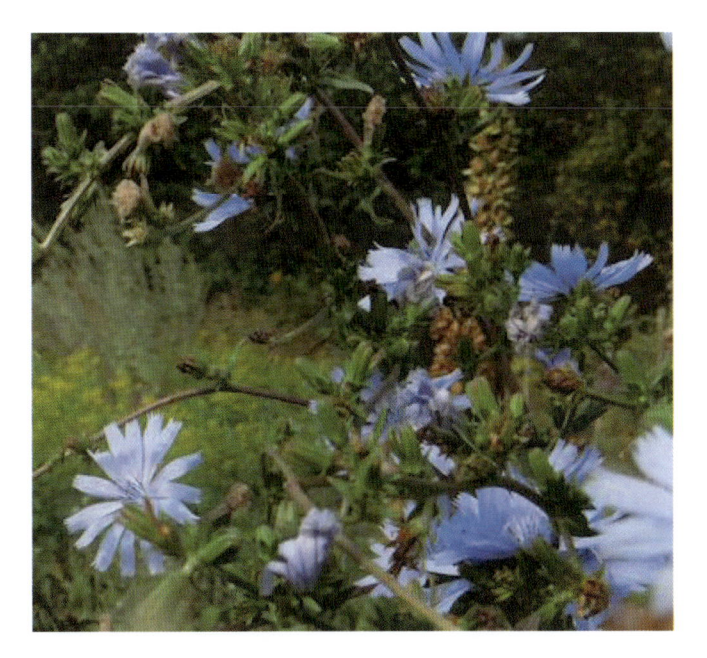

Keywords: letting go, stuck, breaking patterns, ancestral, generational, clarity, resistance, conditioning.

Indications: this essence works hard to break through the resistance of generational patterns. Moving away from the psychological defences.

Healing Qualities: *Helen Wards insights. For people who stick to their usual patterns, being locked within their own psychological defences. It helps to guide a different way. It can create new thought processes within the brain. This essence wants to work directly within the mind. Not to change memories or negate the past, but to say new patterns are needed.*

Those patterns that are generational. The clearing that this essence does enables clarity, dissolving the blinkers, helping us to look to the future.

my own journey with Chicory hasn't always been easy. Having had a mother who's a Chicory type in the Bach Remedies.

Clary-sage

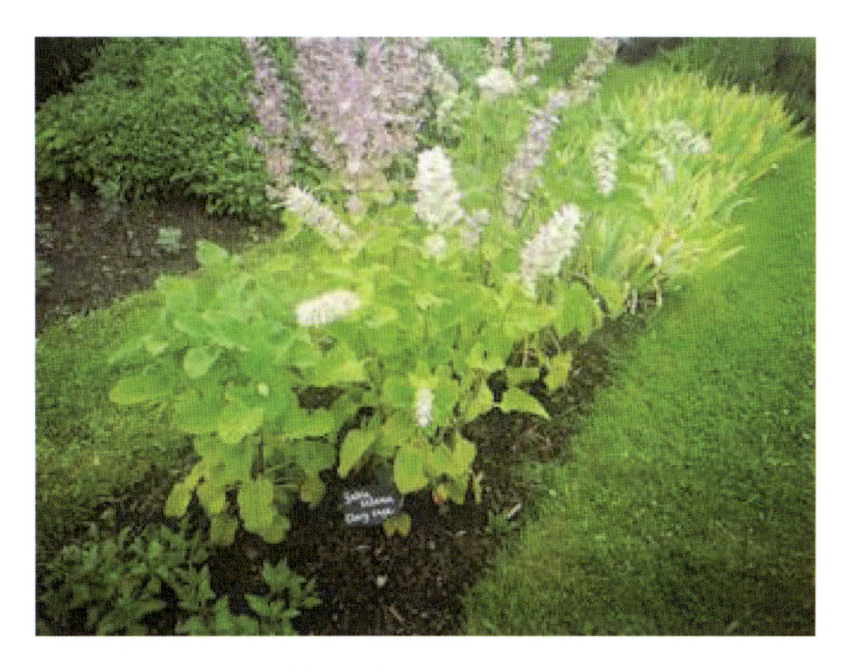

Keywords: adaptability, calmness, inner guidance, wisdom, Transitions, labour, settles, chaos

Indications: Lungs, chest, Helps receive inner guidance from inner knowing. Helps with changes and brings out the wisdom and understanding. For transitions and changes.

Healing Qualities: brings back the meaning to life. Draws wisdom from experience, that are already there. Brings us to a place of acceptance of what life throws at us, in a calm and detached way. Helps find the stillness in the chaos. Helps release can be helpful in letting go as the labour progresses.

Notes: made at the field. Spilled the mother tincture 60ml left added more water. Put it back with the plant touched the flowers. I have never had that happen before.

Cowslip

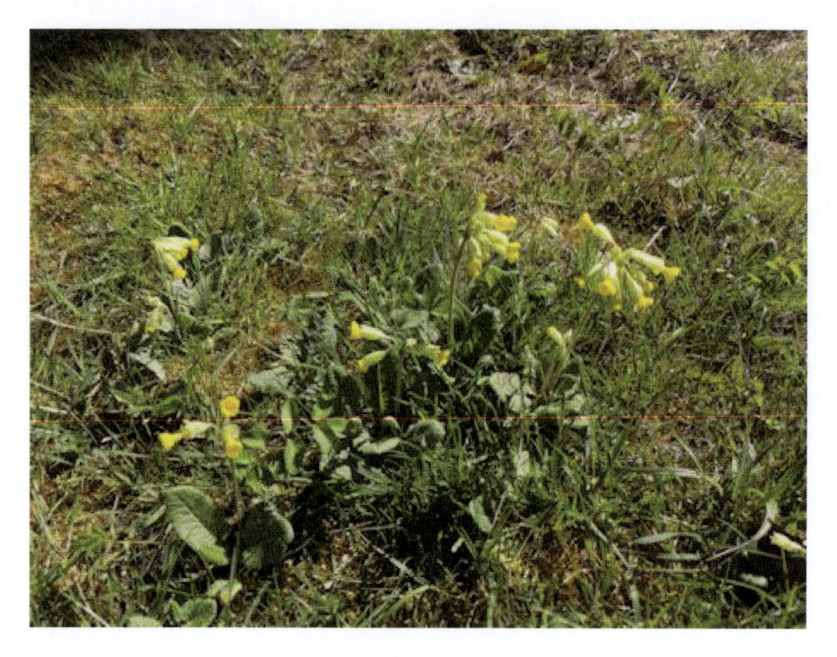

Keywords: prioritising, heart, identity, strength, sadness, heavy hearted, burdened, suppression,

Indications: heavy heart, carrying sadness,

Healing Qualities: the message of this essence is that you are stronger and braver than you know and you are definitely up for the work you were assigned to do. when we have a heavy heart, from carrying burdens that have been placed on you that the family inadvertently placed on you. It enables great release from the burdens that we carry. It releases the sadness from being suppressed. Helping you find your true identity, freeing you up to identify however you wish. This takes you from a place where it has been painful to bee seen, and where a person has been totally misunderstood, within the family

Echinacea

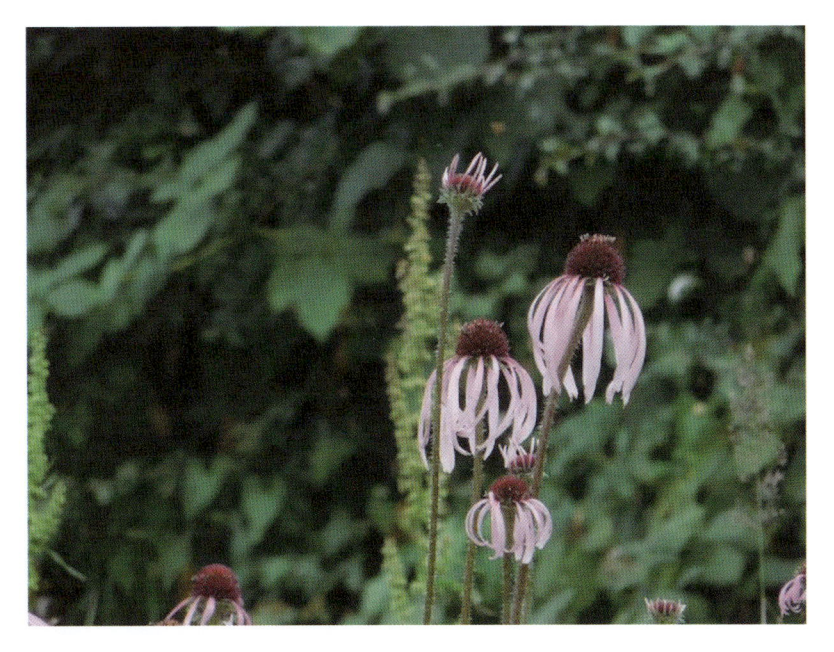

Keywords: integrity, reintegrates, identity, deep trauma, triggers, violence, PTSD,

Indications: Throat Chakra 'Starry Night' was the song that entered my head. Where deep trauma has been experienced maybe impacted on ones identity Where deep rooted trauma has been part of the normal structure and the moral integrity has been shattered. When the stresses of life become too much. Where trauma has been experienced at a very deep level (maybe pre-birth), Echinacea will help to deal with this.

Healing Qualities: Echinacea will strengthen the sense of who you are. Where moral integrity has been shattered from violent acts and situations. It unblocks pathways of communication, realigning and reintegrating leaving a strong knowledge of who you are. Strengthens the sense of identity, helps to maintain a strong sense of self.
use when the stresses of life become too much.

Notes: when this essence was created I went into deep trauma, deep harrowing sobs, gut retching sobs so raw. The following day I felt so raw. I had liberally been wiped out, emptied out. There was also an horrific car accident within the family, fortunately no one was hurt.

this may be combined well with Blackpool mill sea essence.

Great-Burnet

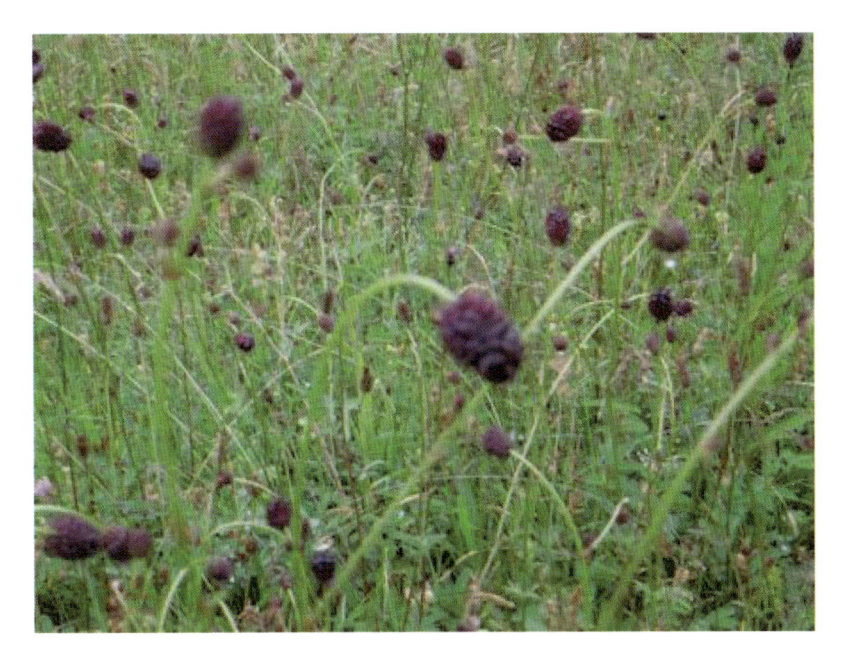

Keywords: calms, sooths, peace of mind, control, heart, conflict, turmoil,

Indications: Base chakra. Heart Chakra. Solar plexus Helps with stomach when it is churning from turmoil. Settles the mind when it is spinning out of control and it won't settle Helps deal with inner conflict, soothing the heart

Healing Qualities: when we are in conflict because we can't control a situation, the reality is that the only thing we are in control of is ourselves, which is exactly what this essence is for, its calming effects will help to bring us to that realisation.
it has a Soothing effect on the heart chakra. Helps when feeling churned up settling you down. When we are beyond stressed, agitated, in a frenzy, it will sooth our frazzled mind, and impact on our emotional and mental body. It sooths the inner turmoil of the mind calming it down when out of control. Helps to reconnect with our inner spirit and guidance.

Notes: started the wrong plant. Conflicted.

Henbane

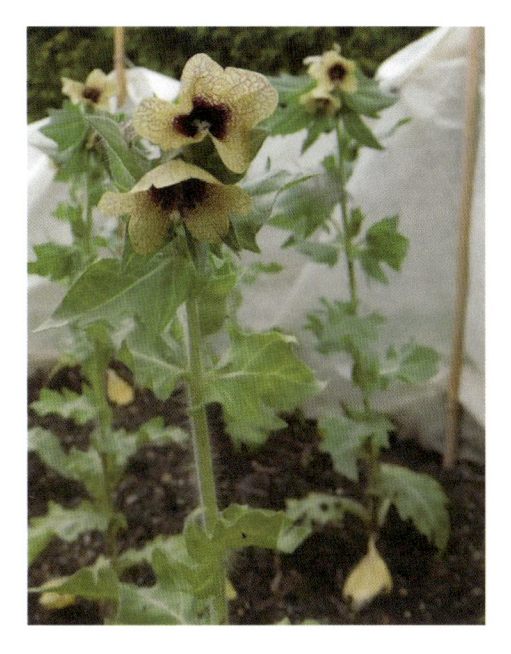

Keywords: Cross-roads, illusion, stability, perspective, death, re-birth, ancestral curses

Indications: 3rd eye, throat, jaw. Heart, When life brings us to a cross-roads, it can help through these transitions.

Healing Qualities: Henbane is for when we are at a crossroads. There are points of change we all go through, these shifts transforming so that we can move forward in life, Changes come in many different ways. Henbane can help us with these times. Whether that is in life or as we transition into Death.

Notes: created on the summer solstice overnight.

I found myself asking questions "what are my opinions" I also felt more sure of myself.

Helen Wards observations, "through this essence we can have more of a sense of the pace and type of life that suits us, so we are not

thrown off course by what suits other people or what our culture/social media imposes on us."

Iris-Germanic

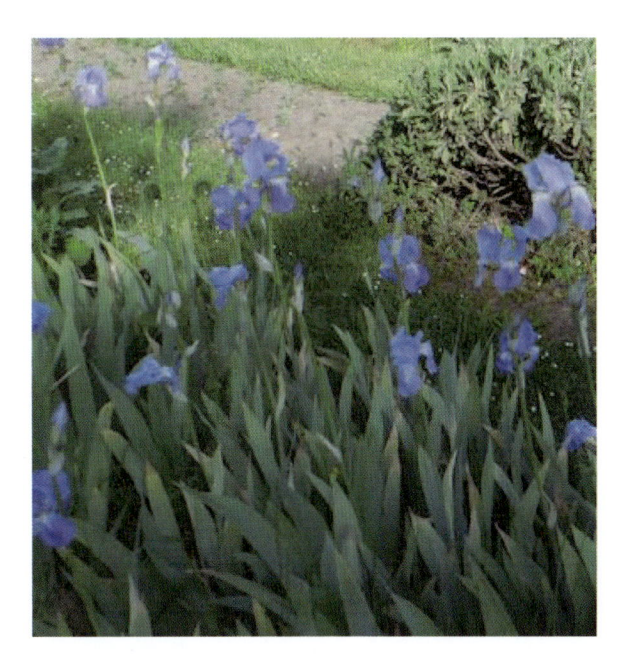

Keywords: personal power, boundaries, creativity, blocked, despair, disgruntled, frustration

Indications: 2nd and 3rd chakra's. it will help to clear frustrations that are blocking our creativity.
Iris enhances the power to our feminine side, male or Female

Healing Qualities: Enhances the power of the feminine, unblocking those blocks to creativity, and ability to express ourselves. Helps with our inspiration.

Iris will help with listening to our inner authority. When we have given too much Iris will help us with draw.

Ivy

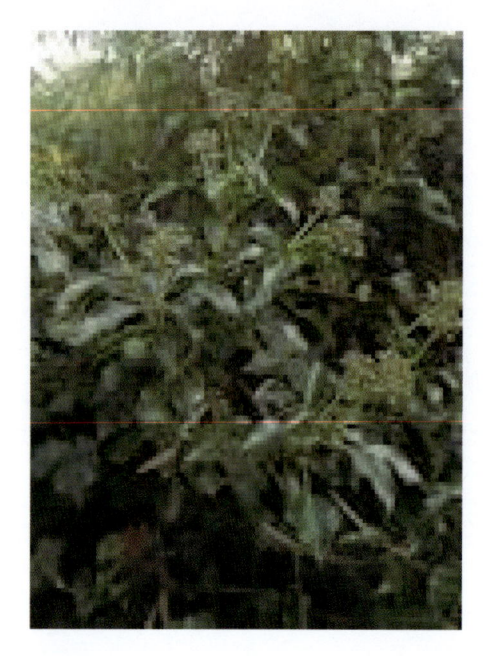

Keywords: connections, resolutions, rhythms, clarity, healthy, resilience, deceptions, disconnected, grounding, roots, obstacles,

Indications: Harnesses the will when we have disconnected - it reconnects, remain to fight another day. it brings in the instinct to survive. Brings what is key for our health.

Healing Qualities:

Good to ground. This essence brings connections that we need to make, it brings the right energies into our awareness. Without the right balance of energies flowing, one finds health harder to access. An essence key to wellness.

This was birthed partly at the field at Weleda and partly from my garden I was guided to bring them together and this was the result .Solutions to problems quickly become apparent, which could have seemed insurmountable, but were quickly resolved, and effectively. i.e. My battery in my car went flat almost straight away 3 lovely guys helped to push start. Other obstacles happened which again were quickly resolved.

Lacy-Phacelia

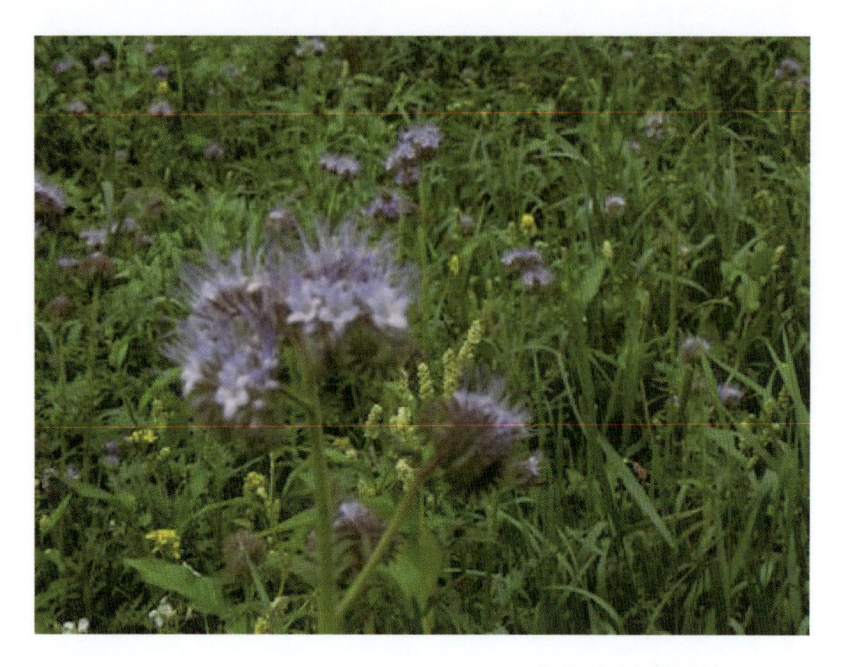

Keywords: convalescing, addictions, resources, trauma, incapacitates, new beginnings, breath, recuperation, nurtured, restores

Indications: this restorative essence, aid us to rehabilitate from life traumas and during times where we need to recover, physically, emotionally, spiritually and mentally.

Healing Qualities: Lacy Phacelia assists us with honouring ourselves accessing our inner resources, breaking those addictive patterns, allowing life to begin again.

Useful when convalescing, from illnesses including virus's that have laid us low, helping with our flow of energy.

Notes: Lacy Phacelia was birthed during the "Harmonic Alignment".

Helen Wards input, It helps earth energy flow, helps us to breath better, helping to restart after traumas that incapacitates.it is also

about allowing life to begin again, that it overcomes paralysis or a sense of deadness inside, that one isn't just looking at life but living it. This life giving essence, nurturing us back to life, also helps us care for others too, so that the well of our love/ compassion doesn't run dry.

this essence connects one to the earth so that the energy can rise up through the various chakra's and go where it is needed. It is very restoring

It is also included in the Recuperation essence.

Lavender

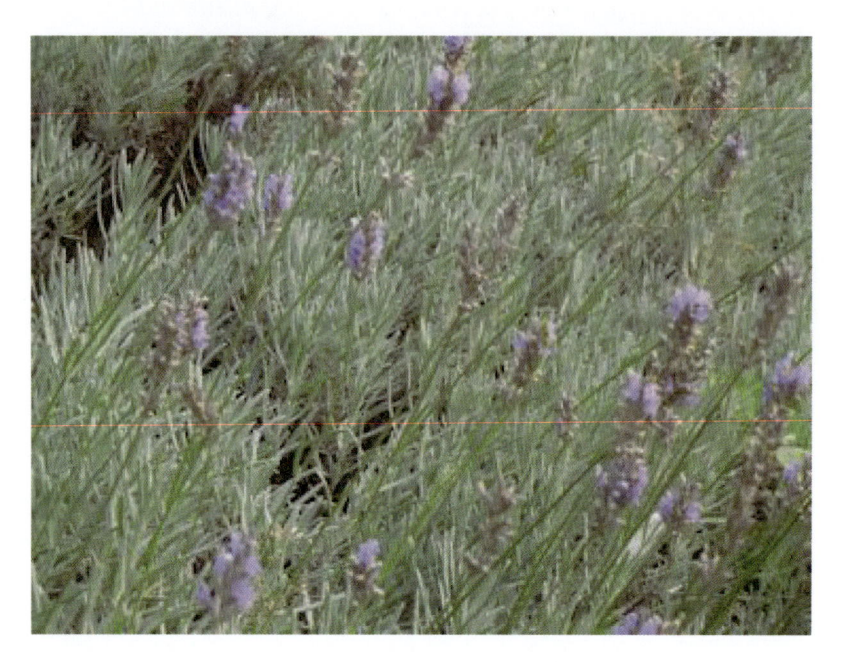

Keywords: frazzled mind, discombobulated, blocked, unemotional, depressed, melancholic, repressed, authentic,

Indications: where the mind is frazzled and you feel in a frenzy. Where we have been cut off from our true nature. For a person who should in their true nature be happy, but just is so caught up with ever present sadness.

Healing Qualities: this can very much be a person who is the joker or comes *Helen Wards this person possibly feels as though they are made of stone, somewhat numb underneath, definitely not in touch, the repression that this person may have encountered, has had an impact.*

Marsh-Mallow

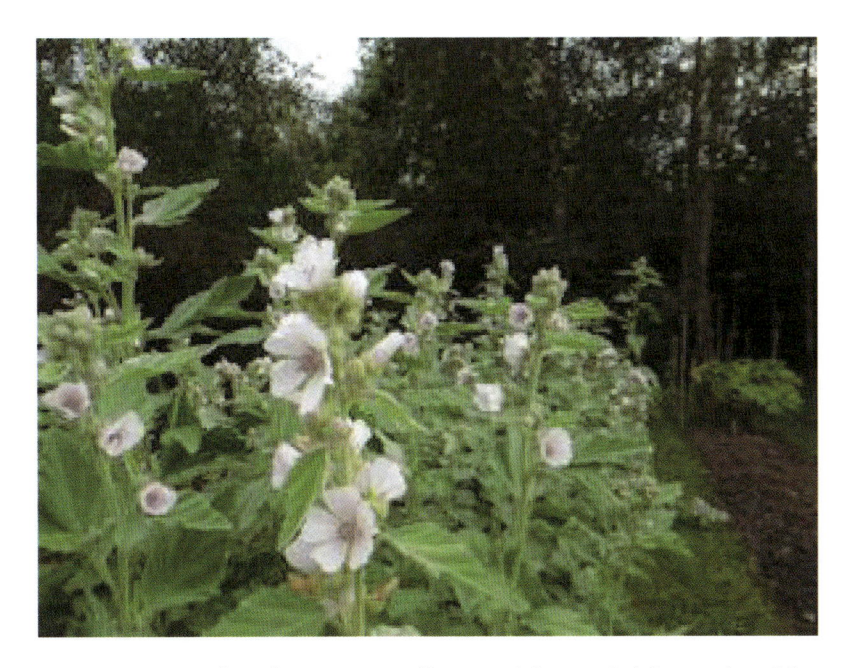

Keywords: calms inner turmoil, transitions, rigidness, hard hearted, Anger, anxiety, worry, letting go, moving on

Indications: crown, 3rd eye, Ears, disconnected from feelings, breaks barriers down. Connects the heart to the lower chakras. Calms the emotional bodies down.

Healing Qualities: every part of this plant has medicinal properties. It was given to babies who were teething, for its analgesic properties. it helps to soften transitions. When in times of turmoil, it will calm and strengthen your resolve. It helps you to let go and move on, It is like receiving a hug. It lifts the spirit.
not long after birthing this beautiful essence, I spent a whole day at Weleda studying Marsh Mallow, the feeling of peace that touched me was simply beautiful. All of the group that were present felt the peace that this beautiful plant.

Mullein

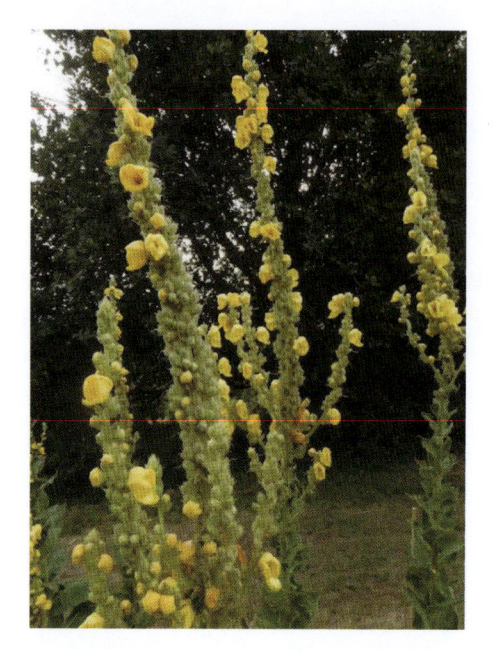

Keywords: Peace, inner light, realigns, inner self, gratitude rebirth, Bruised/battered by life, indecision,

Indications: when life has battered you and you are left feeling raw and venerable

Healing Qualities: lifts you out of raw emotional states. Moving you back into the light into a place of gratitude. Connects you with your own inner light, realigns you back into the light. When you look at this amazing plant you can see the magnificence of the way it literally looks like a beacon. Connects you to your inner light, so you can be your true self.

Poke root

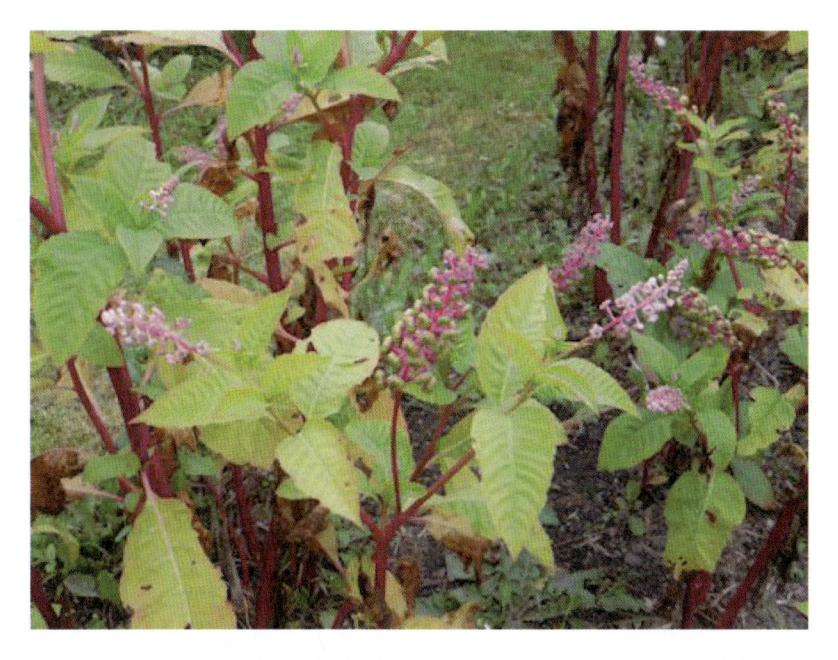

Keywords: male/female balance, self-control, responsibility, strength, security, grounding, balance, anchor, clutter, anger, rage

Indications: heart chakra.
For when anger takes a hold gets a grip. Psychological turmoil may be Indicated.
Clearing out the old and outworn, birthing the new.

Where there has been oppression of the Female.
'Doing', 'Proactive', 'Making things happen'. Strong, steady, balanced. Moving forward.
Where a balances needs to be struck between
Male/Female
Activity/Stillness.
Outward/Inward.
Clearing out the old and outworn, birthing the new.

Healing Qualities: Balanced and harmonious masculine principle. Grounding, balancing, anchoring.

This essence come up when there is deep seated anger, rage that needs to be worked on. For those living too much in their heads, brings them fully into their physical. Conversely, also for those who are strongly in the physical but need to get in touch more with their mental and emotional processes.

Where there are extremes and polarisation and seemingly no middle ground to meet in. Accepting and integrating our masculine and feminine sides. For those who need to let go of the physical – i. e. Accept that it is time to loosen their grip on life and move into spirit... and paradoxically those who are not fully living their lives and are quite ambivalent about being here.

As a herb it is used for Mastitis which gets really angry just like Poke Root.

Notes: *Jan Rose's Insights:*
Doing', 'Proactive', 'Making things happen'. Strong, steady, balanced. Moving forward. Energy coursing up and down legs – Earthing. Drawing strength and energy from the Earth.
Useful when balance is needed e. g. between male and female aspects
(particularly stereotypical extremes such as the macho male or weak and submissive female), work/play, movement/stillness.
Strong masculine energy in hand. 'Doing', 'Proactive', 'Making things happen'. Strong, steady, balanced. Moving forward.
Life. Strength and security. Self control and responsibility.
Heart, Higher Heart and chest area. Space to breathe and be without constraint. Deep breathing – exhaling waste and breathing in Prana.

Energy coursing up and down legs – Earthing. Drawing strength and energy from the Earth.

Useful when balance is needed e. g. between male and female aspects (particularly stereotypical extremes such as the macho male or weak and submissive female), work/play, movement/stillness. Where there are extremes and polarisation and seemingly no middle ground to meet in. Accepting and integrating our masculine and feminine sides. (Might be useful for anyone uneasy with their sexuality or gender, particularly pre-op transsexuals). For those who need to let go of the physical – i. e. accept that it is time to loosen their grip on life and move into spirit… and paradoxically those who are not fully living their lives and are quite ambivalent about being here. Life. Strength and security. Self control and responsibility.

Heart chakra. Space to breathe and be without constraint. Deep breathing – exhaling waste and breathing in Prana. Energy coursing up and down legs – Earthing. Drawing strength and energy from the Earth.

Pulsatilla

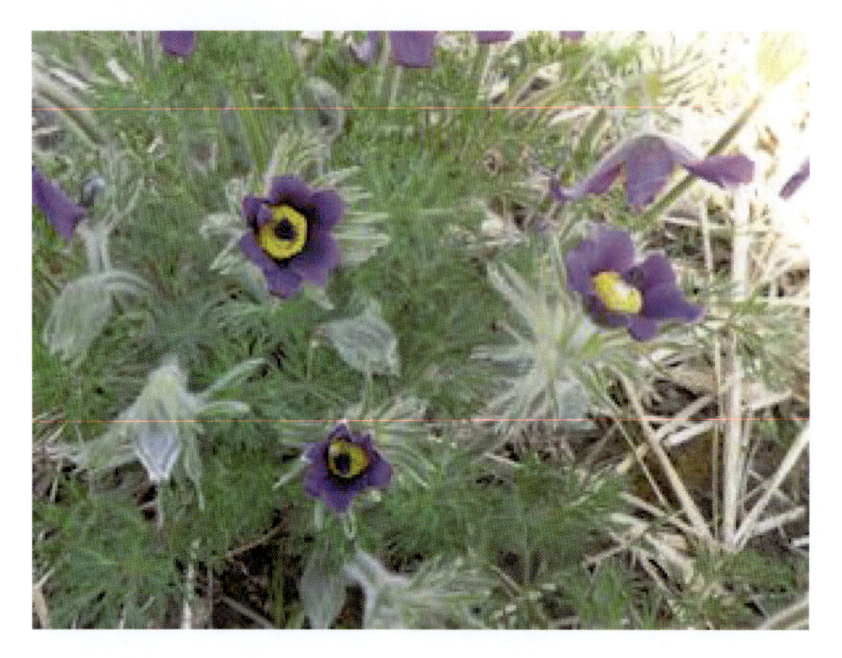

Keywords: weepiness, heart chakra, protector, healer, opener, vulnerable, emotional states, equilibrium,

Indications: heart chakra, changeable states of emotions, weepiness, euphoria. It helps to protect, heal, and open the heart chakra.

Healing Qualities: Pulsatilla balances the vital core strength which enhances inner strength and stability. It brings out gentle feminine side, whilst enhancing and engendering ones inner security and grounds you. helping you recognise and know yourself on a deeper level.
it can enhance deep feelings of love in a very powerful way.
when Pulsatilla was being created, I had an old soul part returned to me. It had been guarded, a long time

Notes: soul part guarded by a Dragon bought back from Ireland.

Rosemary

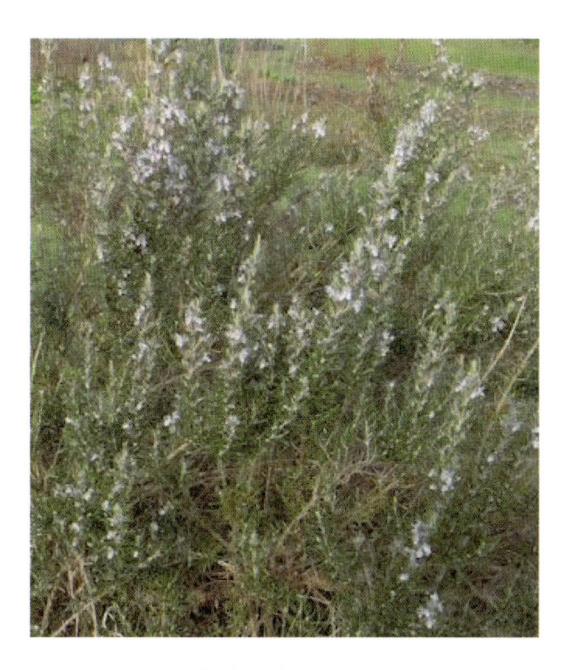

Keywords: clarity, inner peace, protective, balance, power,

Indications: Rosemary is all about remembering who you are and your truth. It brings clarity to the mind and thoughts.

Healing Qualities: Remembering who you are and your truth. This is an essence that helps you stand in your true nature and power. When this takes place it will protect you from the negative opinions of others and challenges.

It became very clear during the period leading up during and after this essence was birthed that it really was about remembering who I was how far I had come. The sentence that kept going through my head was just remember who you are" If you know who you are you can stand in your power.

Notes: There were challenges as this essence was birthed. The words that came to me were Remember who you are.

Scotch-Thistle

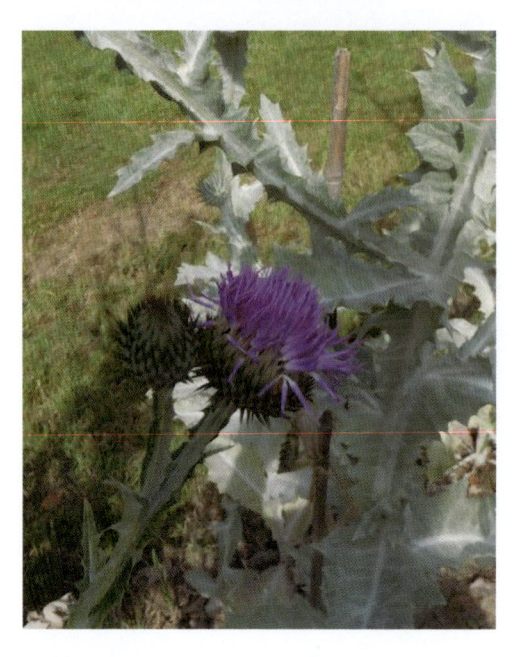

Keywords: courage, supports, calms, strength, grounds, secure, fear, crisis, anxiety, shock, panic,

Indications: This tall strong plant, gives you the courage to breath through the fear and grief. Deals with Fear everyday fears to extreme intense fear, paralysed with fear. Brings in the calmness needed.

Healing Qualities: when you have been rocked to the core, being left feeling totally unstable. It will help deal with crisis. Helps to get in touch and find your inner strength. Keeps you calm and gives the clarity need when your being is in total fear.

Scurvy-Grass

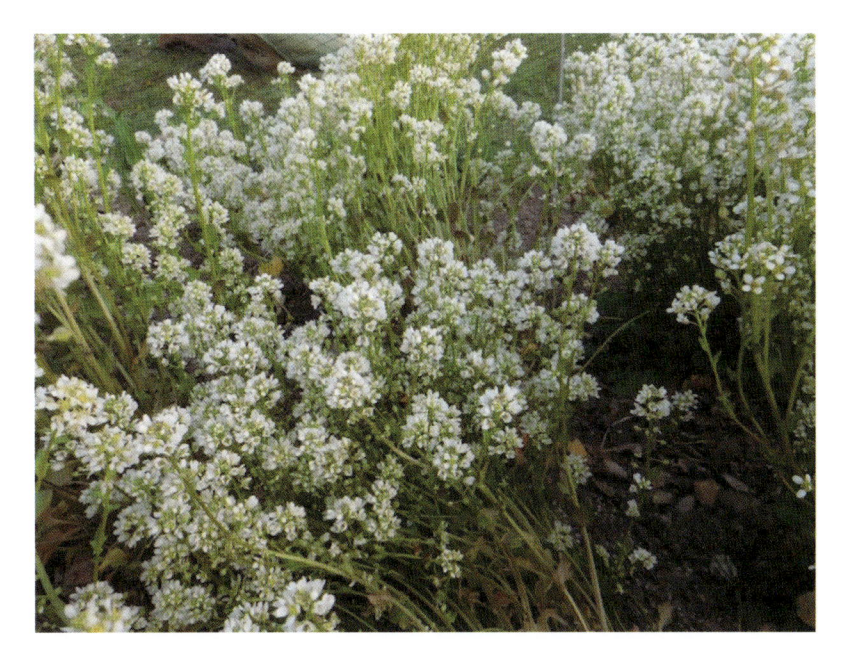

Keywords: acceptance, beauty, value, vulnerability,

Indications: it will help you find the gifts of your experience. What is or has occurred.

Healing Qualities: This essence will help you understand and know your true value. Scurvy grass will help you see and accept your beauty. It helps access the deep parts of your being, helping to gain deeper knowledge and understanding of who you are, helps you to know where you fit.

Notes: made at the field in Ilkeston. Early morning on the 19th I left this essence to be birthed over the full moon from Libra overnight. Collecting and decanting on the 20th after the moon had gone into Scorpio. It was a Good Friday Full moon.

St-Johns-Wort

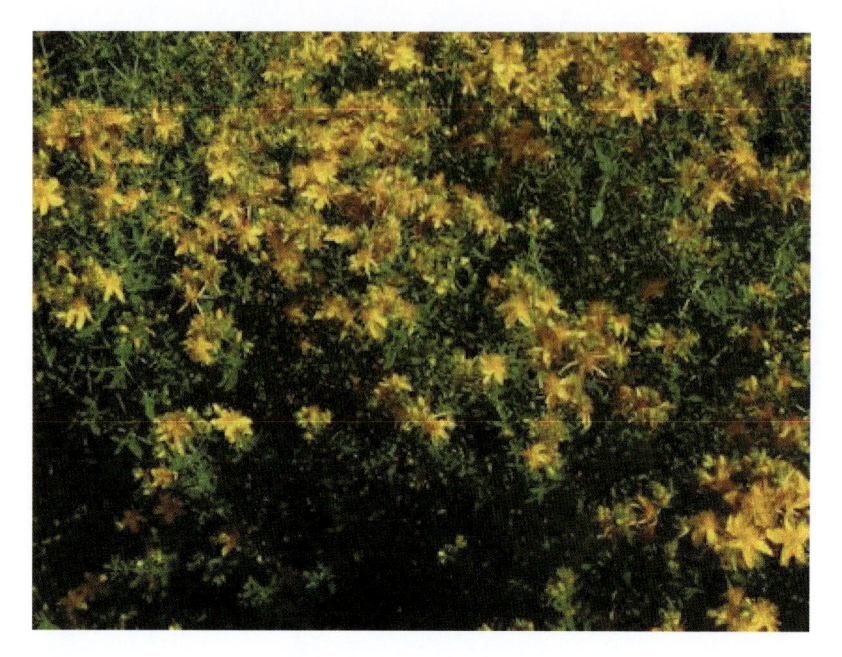

Keywords: peace, strength, optimism, protective, anchor, sleep, anxiety, nightmares, fear, melancholia, depression. vulnerable,

Indications: solar plexus, It reduces fear. Lifts the mood particularly those who struggle with deep melancholia. Brings peace of mind. Deep routed fears. Strengthens the emotional body. Recharges when we have been left depleted. Improves quality of sleep

Healing Qualities: St-Johns-wort is for the sensitive soul. Who can be effected because of their sensitivity. It is a protective essence, which can protect against psychic interference. It can help if a person struggles to keep connection with their body and be more anchored. Acts as an inner light.
Helps deal with those deep routed fears which has resulted in anxiety. Bringing in feelings of strength.

Tobacco

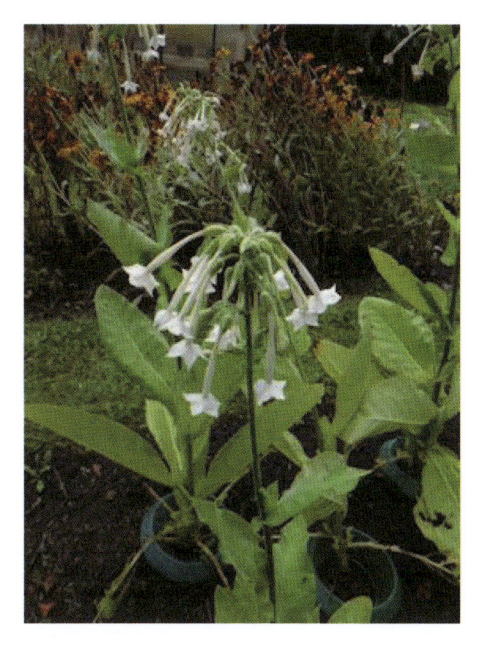

Keywords: grounding, release, shifts, stuck, transformation, envy, possessive, addictions, co-dependency, flexibility, narrow minded

Indications: helps release us from addictions, and systems which don't serve you.

Healing Qualities: for the person who only sees things in black and white. With people who are bigots. Bringing unison within.

Valerian

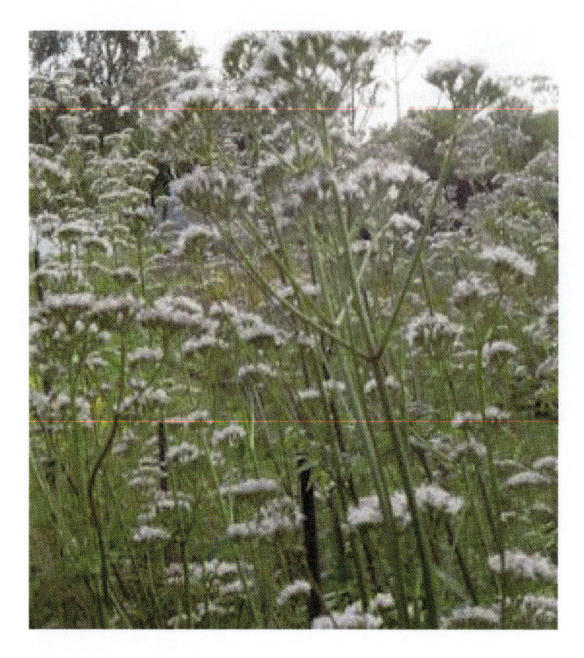

Keywords: sadness, PTSD, shock, Raw, emotions, disconnected, trauma, peace of mind,

Indications: Heart. Brings focus of attention to now. Deals with shock. Brings peace of mind

Healing Qualities: tiny buds very pale pink flowers very sweet smelling. The healing power with-in this plant is amazing. When in shock or PTSD will help bring you back into the present, reconnecting. When you are struggling to function in the world Valerian is a good essence, bringing you back into the present was given to solders during the war for PTSD.
Valium was synthesized from Valerian

Notes: Broke one of the stems. A little girl had an accident. A small portion of her little finger got chopped off. Every one really shook up. This essence was made at the Field.

Vipers-Bugloss

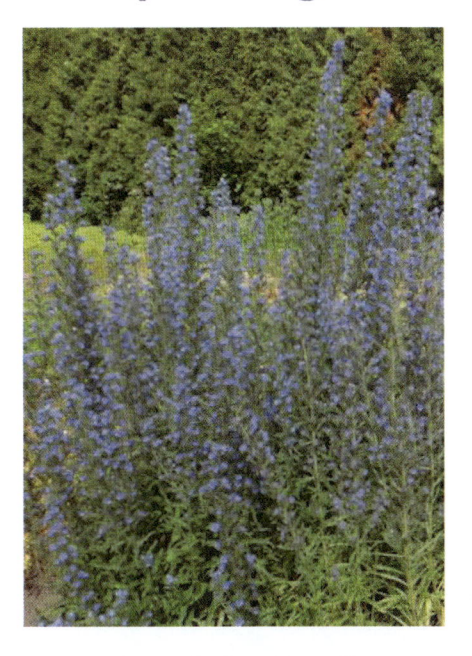

Keywords: victim mentality, communication, pattern breaker,

Indications: throat chakra, pattern breaker. This powerful essence helps to break those destructive patterns. Can help to release us from victim mentality that is ingrained even from childhood. Where negative words have been used in a powerful way as a destructive force.

Healing Qualities: whist in the process of this being created I got bitten on the throat, this indicated it was something to do with the throat Chakra and how we communicate. It was also produced on the solar eclipse.
communication can be a hard the power of words we use can have a huge impact. Vipers bugloss helps us express ourselves in a much more effective and constructive way.
Internal dialogue can be just as damaging, Vipers Bugloss helps with how we internalise our and thoughts in a positive light. Which in turn creates positive experiences and new patterns of behaviour.

Yarrow

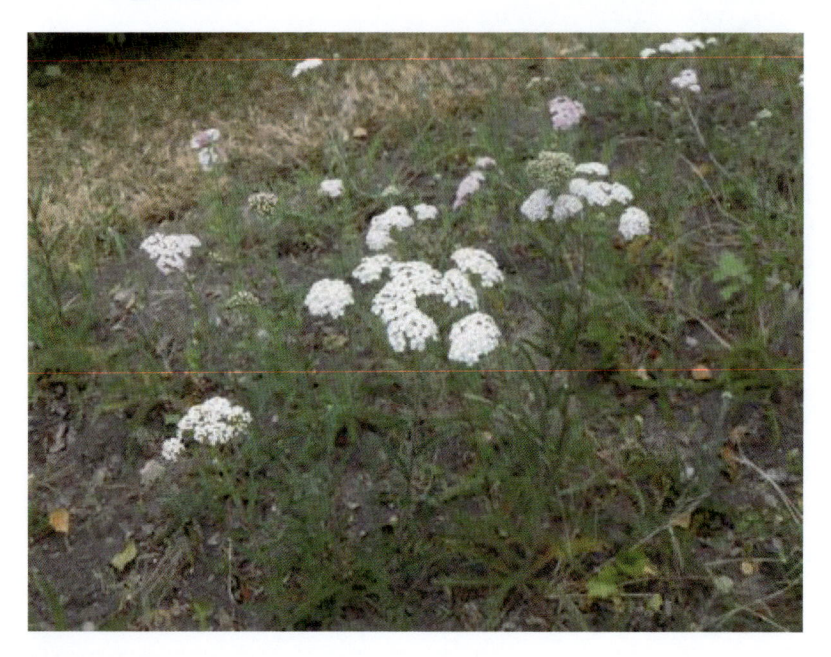

Keywords: chakras, trauma, protective

Indications: childhood trauma, protects and strengthens the aura. It will stop the Aura leaking.
Ideal for therapists to help remain impartial or the parent when they are dealing with their child's trauma or pain.

Healing Qualities: Yarrow, stops the flow of emotional energy from old outdated patterns to new ways of being. Helps deal with childhood traumas. Aids you with protection when you have witnessed or experienced traumas.
if you are working on certain chakras then it will enhance this work and balance those centres.
lots of my own childhood memories came flooding back.

Notes: decanted in vodka. Lots of childhood memories came flooding back

Fungus Essences

Turkey-Tail-Bracket-Fungus

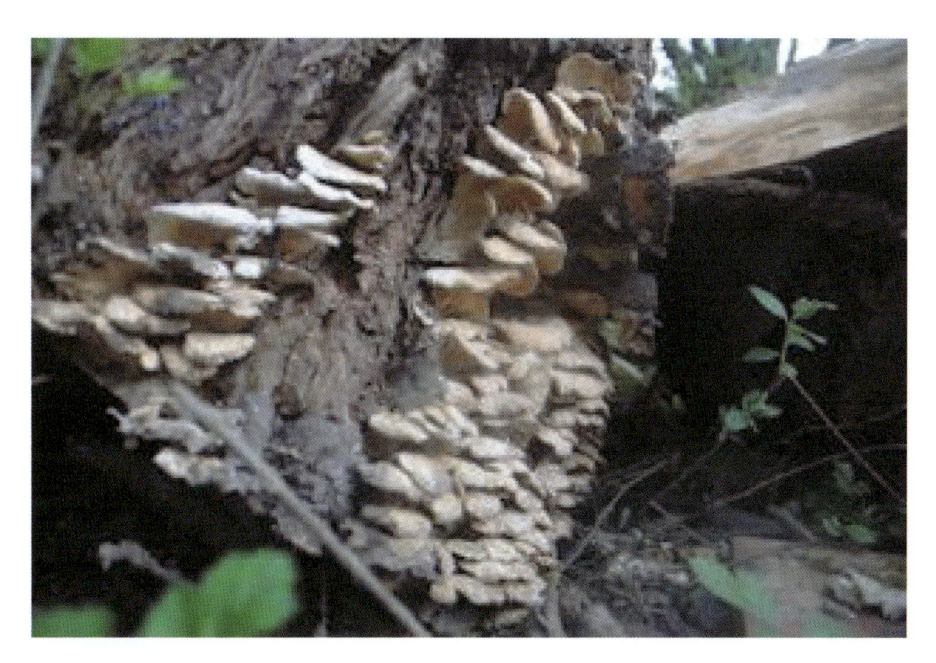

Keywords: soul parts, emotional /energy cleanser, protective. inner-child, nourishing,

Indications: Helps clear emotional scar tissue,

Healing Qualities: Helps clear emotional scaring, brings soul parts back,

Jan Stewarts insights. Fiercely protective essence that will ward off even the darkest energies.it is also nourishing and in particular, effects feelings of safety, support and encouragement for the inner child. It will also seek out and help balance areas and issues that need to be addressed during periods of recovery from trauma which makes since as it is included in Recuperation combination.

Notes: included in the recouperation combination. Trametes Versicolor or Coriolus versicolor.
People take this for immunity, people who have had chemotherapy take it as a tincture.

lots of things were missing as this essence was being created. I also had a mild headache and sore throat.

Gem Essences

Basalt

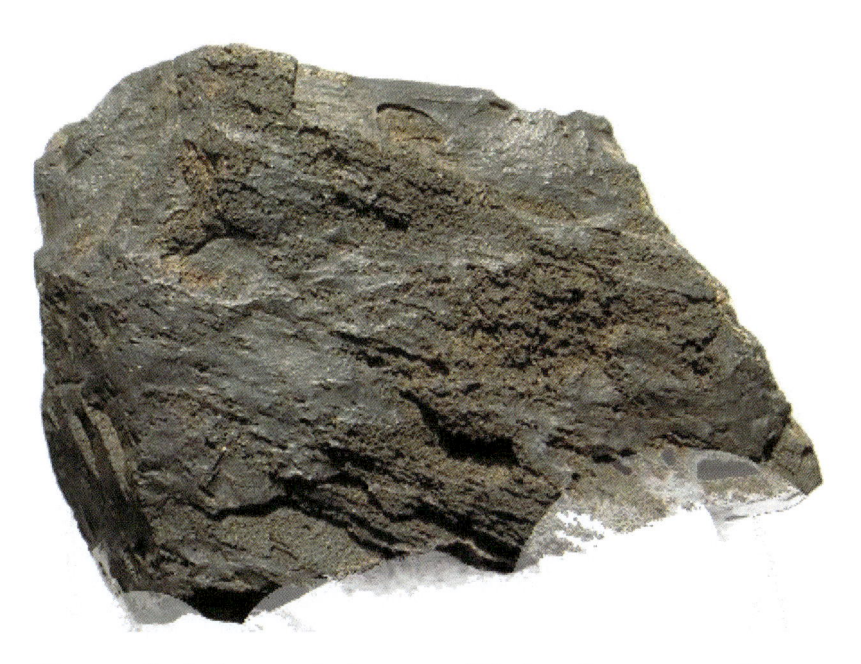

Keywords: balance, clarity, consolidation, focus, grounding, procrastinate, prioritise, feeling, seeing clearly, manifesting, taking action, achieving, psychic abilities

Indications: Heart chakra, Solar Plexus chakra, Soles of Feet chakra's 3rd Eye chakra.
This essence is great for manifestation ideas into reality. For prioritising. Brings in Balance. Feelings, seeing clearly , taking action, achieving. Good if you have Psychic abilities.

Healing Qualities: Bringing ideas, inspiration and spirituality down to Earth. Good for when someone has a lot of different 'irons in the fire' and needs to focus on just one exclusively so that they can be successful.

Useful to take when someone is full of ideas and schemes but cannot ever make them real or workable e. g. The New Ager who has spent 10 years talking in detail about how he is going to take a trip to India 'One day' and the various overland routes and transport that could be used etc. but who has barely made it out of his home town in all of that time. This essence would be good for getting him to shift his perception so that his daydream becomes a realistic goal, and to form a workable plan of action (e. g. pricing up the cost of travel, finding work, setting up a savings account etc.). Useful for procrastination. Turning ideas into reality. Brings in balance.

Good when someone has a lot of different 'irons in the fire' and need to focus on just one exclusively , so that they can be successful.

Obsidian

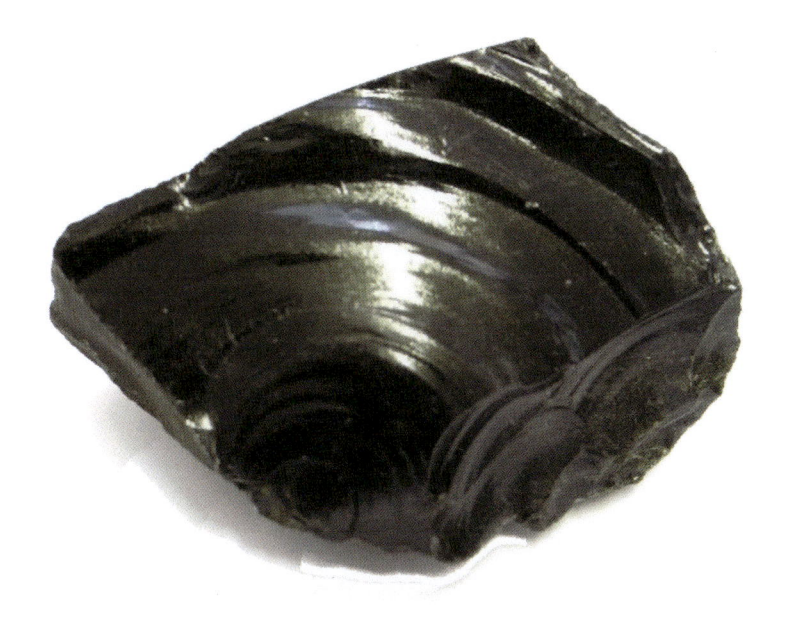

Keywords: deflection, detachment, protection, fortitude, strength, perceptiveness, tension, psychic attack,

Indications: Putting things into perspective Standing back. Cold Detachment. Solar Plexus shielding. 'Seer's shield'.
Reflects and deflects back any psychic or astral level attack.
Good if you want or need to remain unreadable.

Healing Qualities: *Jan Rose's insight*
Use before any high level spiritual work or when under or at risk of psychic attack.
Good when going into any psychically disturbed area (e. g. where murder, black rituals have occurred) – nothing can attach to you. Helpful when you are in a group where you are at risk of attack or interference from another member (e. g. some development circles). When you need to be 'unreadable' by anyone else. Where unhealthy attachments need to be severed in an efficient and dispassionate manner. It brings in strength and fortitude.

This always come up when someone is being subjected to psychic attack and will protect in a strong way.

It promotes strength and fortitude. Helps put things into perspective. Good to use when the moon is changing.

Pearl

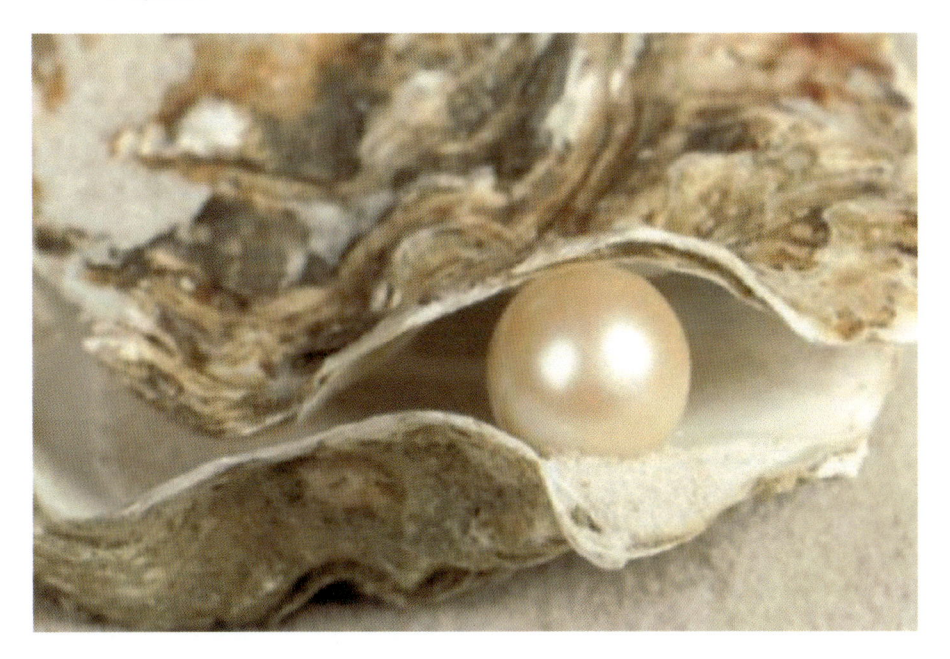

Keywords: feminine power, wholeness, completion, soul retrieval, power,

Indications: 3rd eye, heart chakra, sacrum chakra
Working with the grit and dirt making something of lasting worth.
This is good when we are working with issues that we are not comfortable with.
It will also protect our soul from feeling the pain of others.
For journey to wholeness and completion.

Healing Qualities: The ability to go back in time and find a place where you were happy and carefree - i. e. the true person, the person you truly are by nature and were always meant to be.
Able to access the good times and bright spots in your life, even though memories of tough times may have intruded and inched them out. If you can regain these good times from your past and the resulting positive feelings from them, you can bring them forward into the now.

Wholeness. Completion.
Maybe good for soul retrieval work?

For working with the grit working with the dirt. Making something of lasting worth. Pearl is about heart to heart energy, bringing strength to the heart chakra. It's about loving the self.

Mother of pearl helps you step into your power. Pearl has a creative feminine beauty.

Notes: *Jan Rose's insights*
Firm and steady, travels up the arm to the heart. A burst of sun. Heart. Sacral. Great joy. 'All that is'. A bright sun with visible flares coming off it. Incredibly bright. A young blond haired woman, smiling and happy (Julie when younger?). The light is so intense that is difficult to see clearly.

Channelled Essences

Bridging-the-Gap

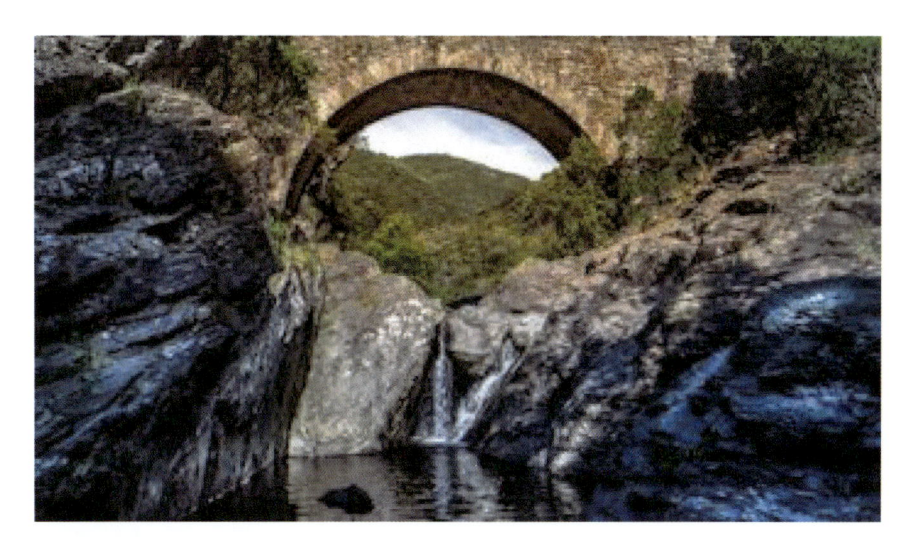

Keywords: transitions, regroup, stuck, unblocks

Indications: helps us to regroup, and move forward when stuck.

Healing Qualities: I was given the name of this essence before, and then channelled the energy that came through. Helps to reconnect to ourselves. I was able to use it to help a lady in a coma, it helped her to journey back to herself. Helen's insights really confirmed this, she talks of a long slumber.

Notes: As the energy came through I could see an ancient dragon, also lots of pearls. At the time around this essence was birthed a close friend was in a coma, this essence helped give me easy access and helped me to connect with her even though she was thousands of miles away. I could see her in a corridor she didn't want to be here. I gave her a pearl also connected to her in hospital and gave her another, pearl which helped her to reconnect back to herself.

Helen wards insights, This is a wake up call for the psyche. It is an essence of transition. Good to take when any process has got stuck. I feel like a sleeper in a cave waking from a long slumber. This essence is good for transitions

---

Galactic-Configuration

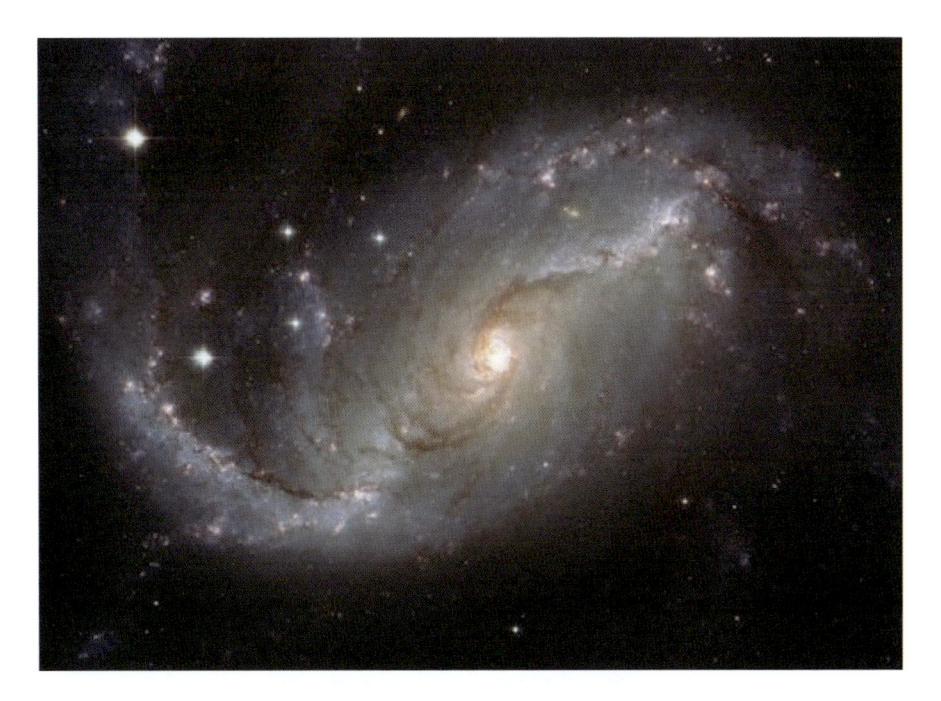

Keywords: lost soul, hold steady, safe, grounds, chaos, anchor,

Indications: Anchors you back in your body. Holding you steady whilst the changes within the earth happens. It helps you feel safe.

Healing Qualities: When I was given the first part of the Name of this essence I got "Galactic. After channelling this essence I got configuration *Karen Read "Age of Aquarius" was the song the came through.* If you read the words to that song it really enables you to understand this essence.

When I read the word to this song it was totally in keeping with this essence, as more and more things a exposed this essence will enable you to deal with the seemingly world in chaos, it will help us to incorporate the new world view, holding us so that we can feel safe.

Helen Ward reminds you of who you are. It brings you back home to yourself. Could be called 'A lost soul essence.

Notes: this was channelled just before the spring equinox on the 18/3/21

Rainbow-Warrior

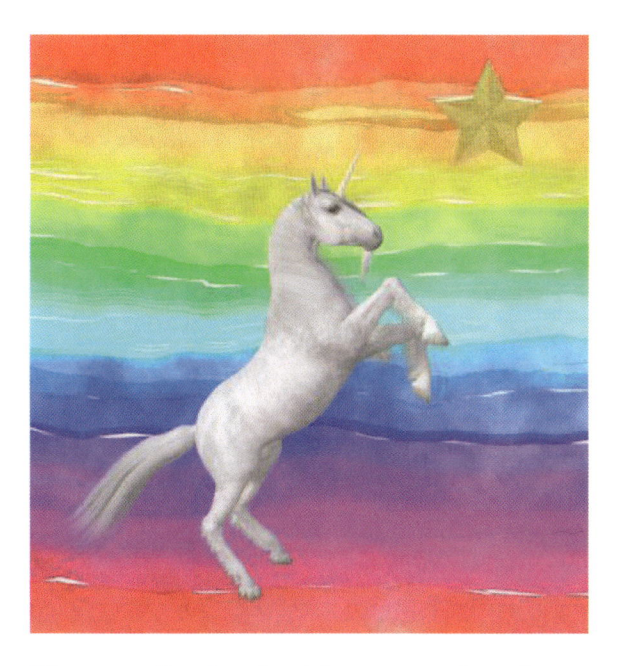

Keywords: destiny, home, authentic, peace,

Indications: Way home, being our authentic self.

Healing Qualities: Two songs were gifted to me the first was "Rainbow Warrior" the second song was "Would you like to swing on a star". This essence is all about being who we are, not succumbing to outside influences. It can help us to see what we can do in the world. Being the Star in your life and shining out in the world, so that we can meet our destiny.

This essence was channelled, as it was downloaded it, I saw a beautiful pure white Unicorn Called "Rainbow Warrior" I was given the name of this essence prior to channelling it. The songs came latter, and the other information followed.

Some information came from Helen Ward. When I re-read the words to "Would you like to swing on a Star" this confirmed the insights Helen's had, she saw lots of swirling rainbows, rainbow painted flags, a dove, who gave the message that they were the emissary for peace. Another name that would have been appropriate would have been 'The Way home'

flags, a dove, who gave the message that they were the emissary for peace. Another name that would have been appropriate would have been 'The Way home'

Seaweed Essences

Bifurcaria

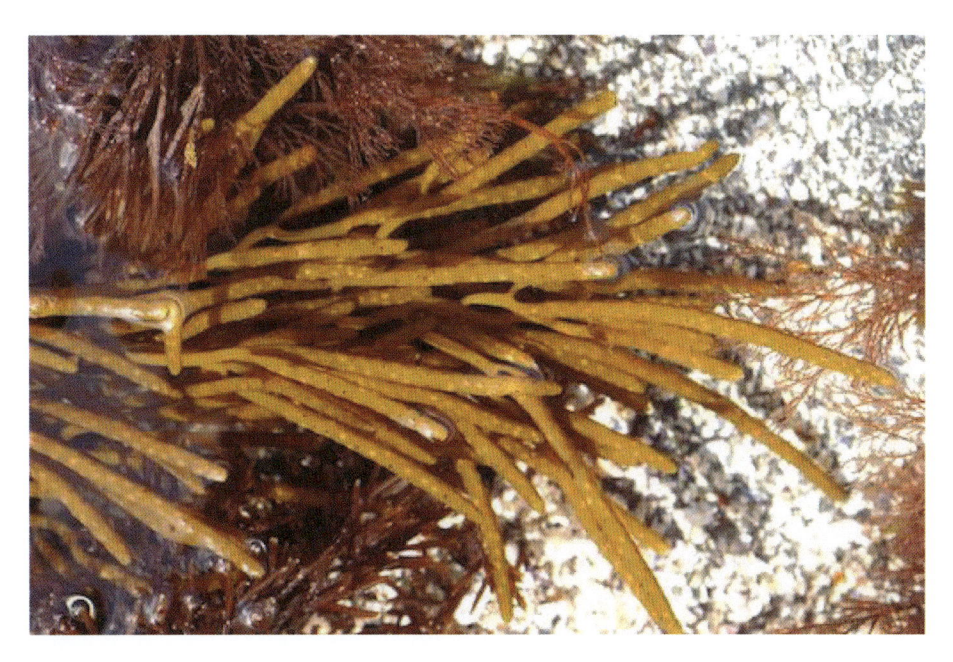

Keywords: life tensions, stress, conflict, relationships, unsettled, confusion, objectivity, clarity, resolution, unties knots, problems solver, aligns, Akashic records, stress, peace

Indications: 3rd eye and what that balances. Aligns the emotional and etheric body.
This is a great essence for those suffering from high tensions, stress, confusion and conflict in relationships. It helps with resolution of personal issues and greater fulfilment. Bringing Peace and clarity.

Healing Qualities: It brings clarity to our senses and peace to our emotions to give us real insight into relationships. This essence helps us appreciate exactly where you are in the moment, making the most of it.

Helping make sense and untie the tangles and knots in relationships and situations.
It is excellent for seeing what is really there, not what you expect to see. It helps to get rid of preconceived ideas. Looking deeper, going beneath the surface. It brings with it clarity and peace
It helps to bring compassion to the soul.

It brings resolution of personal issues and greater fulfilment.
This essence would be useful for those who have difficulty settling – whether in a new place, job or into life on Earth. It is about being still and appreciating exactly where you are now at this precise moment in time and making the most of it.

Erik Pelham's additions
Aligns the emotional and Etheric bodies. It brings clarity to our senses and peace to our emotions to give real insight into relationships. It aids objectivity about our feelings and about ourselves generally, so we can really assess our relationships and be discerning about them.
So many people are in a state of confusion about their relationships and consequently themselves, and this can lead to a lot of unhappiness and wasted time and effort. By bringing real emotional clarity and sharpness to our senses we can see and assess ourselves in a particular relationship situation more easily.

When emotional turmoil and confusion is reduced, deep feeling of peace can come and we gain greater overall wellbeing. As feelings, thoughts and senses come into line we can be much more integrated and more productive with our efforts. This in turn leads to fulfilment and a sense of achievement.

It promotes strength and fortitude.
Helps put things into perspective.

Good to use when the moon is changing

Notes: I often see a sea horse, (guardian) that works on a soul star level, sea horses operate at a very high vibrational level. They are carriers of information.

Jan Rose's insights
Very murky and dark on the bottom. Quite scary. Want to ascend back into the light. Feet touch the bottom. Force myself to stay there and look around. When I keep still the silt settles and the murkiness clears.

I can only see a little way but can see the wreck of an old wooden ship. Wonderful shoals of brightly coloured fish swim through and around it. It seems to have become a sanctuary for all sorts of creatures, all living within and around it. It was amazing watching all the various creatures making their home there and living alongside each other. I was sorry to leave them and return to the surface.

Blackpool Mill

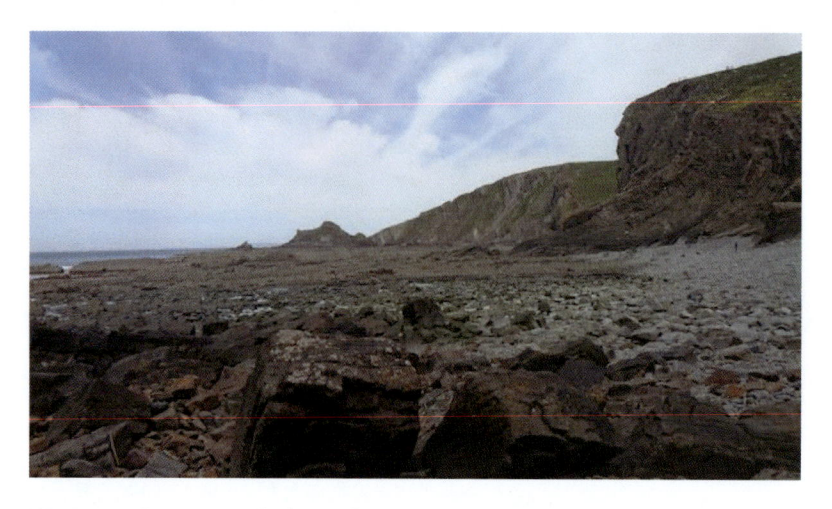

Keywords: overwhelm, cleanser, de-clutter, space, perspective, overwhelm, time out, mental congestion

Indications: Clears your energy field leaving you with a sense of space. It is also a great space cleanser. Helps you to de-clutter, not only the physical, spiritual, mental but also the emotional. Clears the head of clutter helps put things into perspective. Can be used in a cleansing spray.

Healing Qualities: Time away from the rat race. Cuts out and eradicates the negativity. Clears the energy field. The sentence that came to mind was "leaves you with the Golden silence." It helps you get a better perspective.

Notes: when this essence was being created it was a beautiful day we went down to the beach and felt so calm, everything was still. it took me ages to realise what this essence was about, one evening whilst working with a group, I suggested we take a look at "Blackpool mill", I didn't say what it was. One of the group said before taking it their head was full of clutter after they found that their head was empty. All of us had the same experience. One of the group said "leaves you with the golden silence. It did make me smile no wonder I had struggled with this essence. Looking back to the day it was birthed that is exactly what my experience was just perfect. Like all the other sea essences this wanted to be added into the combination.

Caherdaniel Bladderwrack

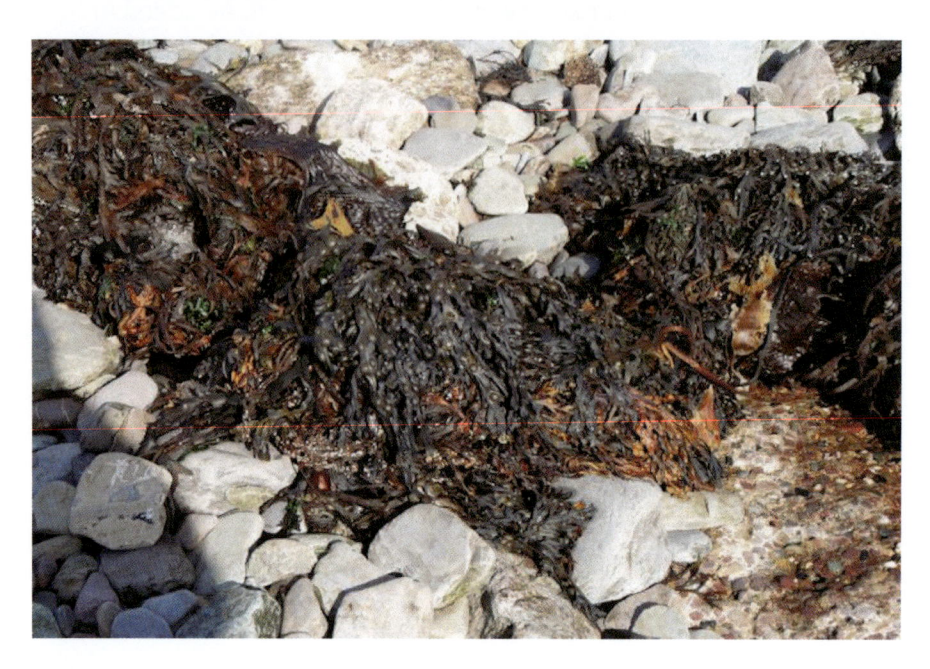

Keywords: chaos, fear, turmoil, safe, sooths, calms

Indications: 3rd eye, throat chakra, base chakra
Eye in the storms of life. When faced with emotional turmoil it will helps to smooth and soothe. Grounding your energy.

Healing Qualities: This essence will hold you in a place where you feel safe. When we are encountering challenges that life presents it will help us feel safe.
it is proving to be a really useful essence for people encountering storms in their life, holding them and keeping them centred and strong.

Notes: This essence I made in 2016 right on the west coast of Ireland in the middle of Storm 'Ophelia' at no give time was I afraid. We were staying in a caravan 20 yard from the beach. Totally unafraid I just felt calm and held.

Corallejo - Halimeda tuna

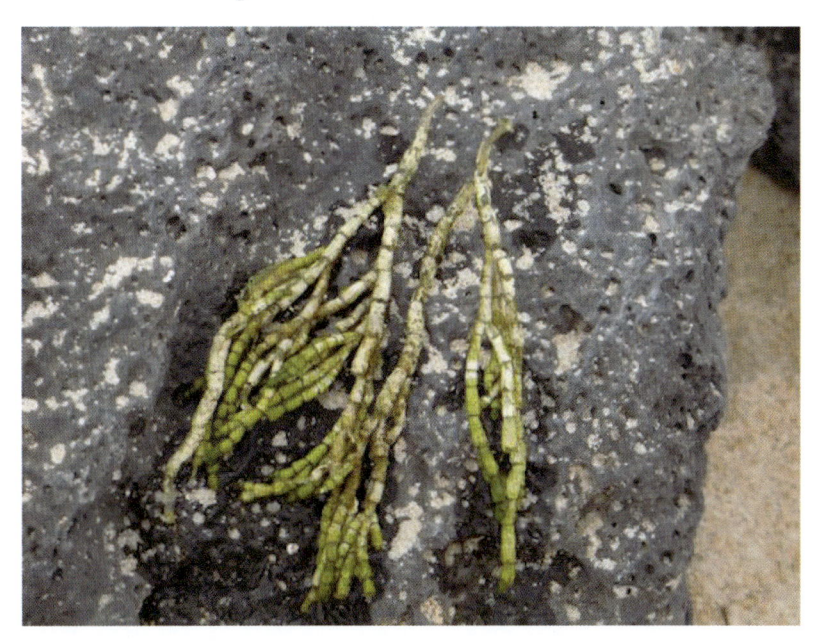

Keywords: toxic, relationships, environment, land, toxic, energy

Indications: Lightens the load. This essence is about disconnecting from toxic relationships. Will emotionally balance a toxic environment helps to clear.

Healing Qualities: This essence clears on many levels, it is for toxicity clearing toxic relationships, environment, and objects. It will help to disconnect from difficult emotions behind toxic relationships.

Notes: When I made this essence, the water turned bright green, its appearance was classically toxic green. Halimeda tuna seaweed is an algae that comes in various shapes - this one I found in Corallejo

Coralline

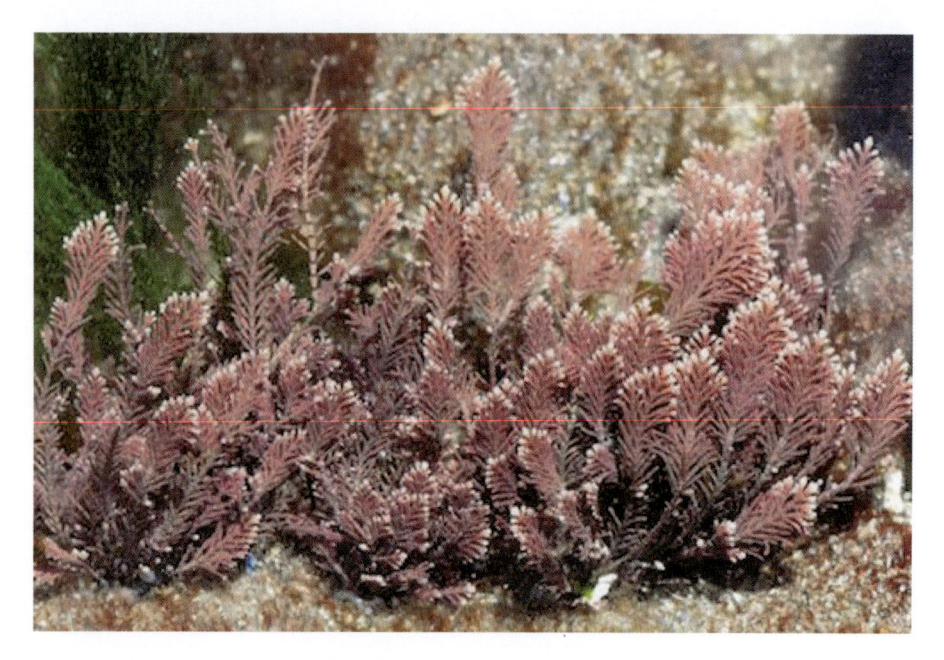

Keywords: chakras, rebooting, rebuilds, restores, strength, clarifies, distress, stress, empower, flow

Indications: 3rd eye chakra
Restores proper rhythms and flows.
Good for people and animals who are out of balance through illness or stress.

Good for land which has been carved up, disrespected or polluted. Helps restore the flow. If your feeling distress this essence will restore the balance.

Healing Qualities: Where proper flow has been interrupted, and needs to be restored. For restoring flow into and out of the home. Where a road system has been altered and a new flow needs to be established. For encouraging water to flow in helpful ways e.g. away from a house.

Where sea walls and defences and harbours have altered the natural flow of the tide, helps the water to settle to the new ways.

This empowering essence gives strength and clarity. It helps to distress. When there is little or no balance it restores brings strength particularly where there has been illness, helping to rebuild from a deep level.

Notes: *Jan Roses insights*
Ears covered by someone else's hands. Temples. Can feel the movement of tides.

Circuit of the body – up the front of the face, over the head, down the back and then up the front of the body. Rhythmic tide flowing around this body circuit.

Derrynane Kelp

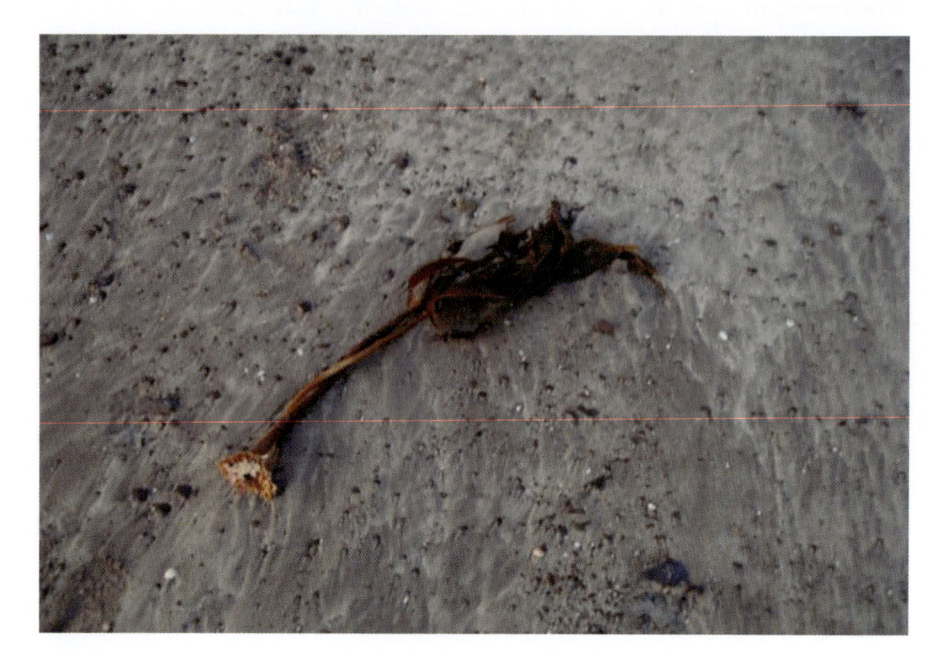

Keywords: irritation, anger, energy protection,

Indications: This is an essence helping when we are irritated or for issues with anger.

Healing Qualities: When we are irritated, or angry with out good reason, this is an essence that will settle the emotions.

Notes: During the time this essence was making I became really irritated to the point of anger. There was no reason other than I was linking into what this essence was about.

Iona

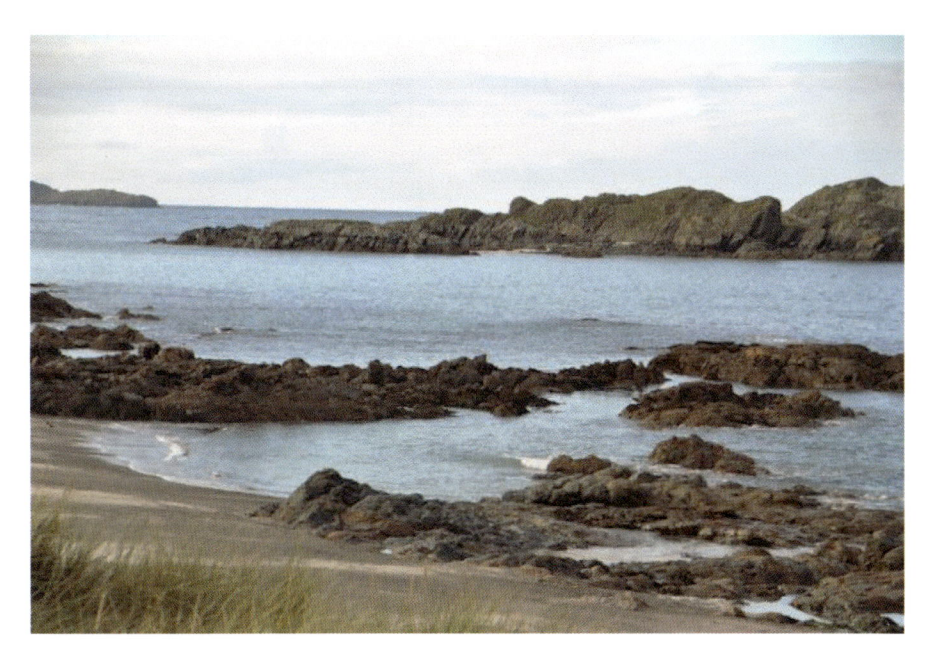

Keywords: dark night of soul, deep melancholia, disconnection, aloofness, mental anguish, lonely, depression, melancholia, recharge, element rebalancer, discernment, reconnects, calm, invigorates

Indications: It helps you too live life real.
This essence recharges, rebalances. It will both calm and invigorate as needed. Balances the elements within us, strengthening those that are weak, calming those that are overactive, particularly in the head.

Healing Qualities: It helps with mental tension, anguish. Where there is inner torment, 'Dark night of soul' deep melancholia. Bringing us back to balance. When we are balanced and whole we are enabled to sense and touch spirit and bring it fully into our lives. It brings us back in touch with the natural world. It also works well on balancing land too.

Jan Rose's insights
Where there is depletion, overpopulated, and built up places where spirit and the wild seem to be keeping a low profile, helps to bring back that natural presence. This essence helps to reconnect. Helps to ground.

An essence of and for life in all its mood, seasons, phases and tempestuous beauty. This is a big essence, a melding of sea and sky Wind and Earth. It has a strong mix of these elements, each recognisable with a distinct identity of their own, but with the capacity to come together and birth between them something far broader and greater in spirit. It is really a natural form of alchemy.

Notes: For this essence I collected a variety of sea weeds, I took them back to Mull, and made it just up from the Sea.

Kefalonia

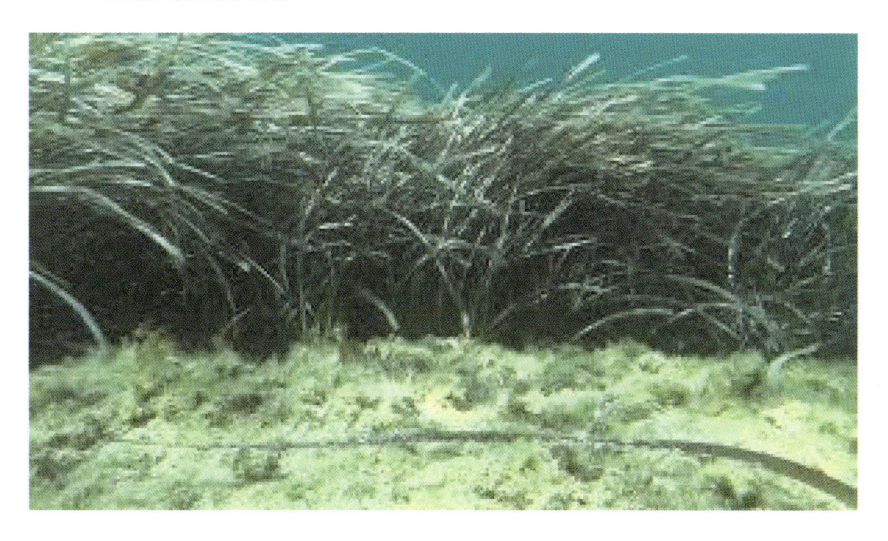

Keywords: purifies, cleanses, thoughts, filters emotions,

Indications: Heart chakra, purity of thoughts and being. Helps get to the heart of the matter.

Healing Qualities: This essence works slowly but very powerfully, really helping to address what is needed. It seems to filter and cleanse.

Kelp

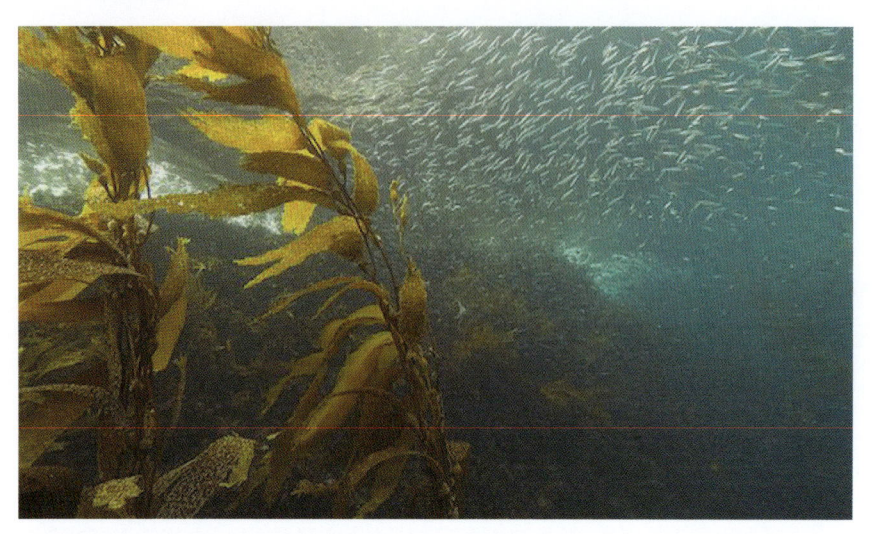

Keywords: focus, faith, change, pattern breaker, trauma, shock, people , animal, land, addictions

Indications: Gentle in the hand. Heart chakra, throat chakra.

This will help gently shift long standing patterns. Brings change gently but effectively.

Healing Qualities: Helps us to have the 'Faith All Will Be Ok'
It is also a good essence for focus

For gently eroding and shifting stubborn and longstanding patterns. For gently effecting change, particularly where there has been great challenges that have left you raw – in land, animals and people. For where 'Less is more'.

Kelp-holdfast

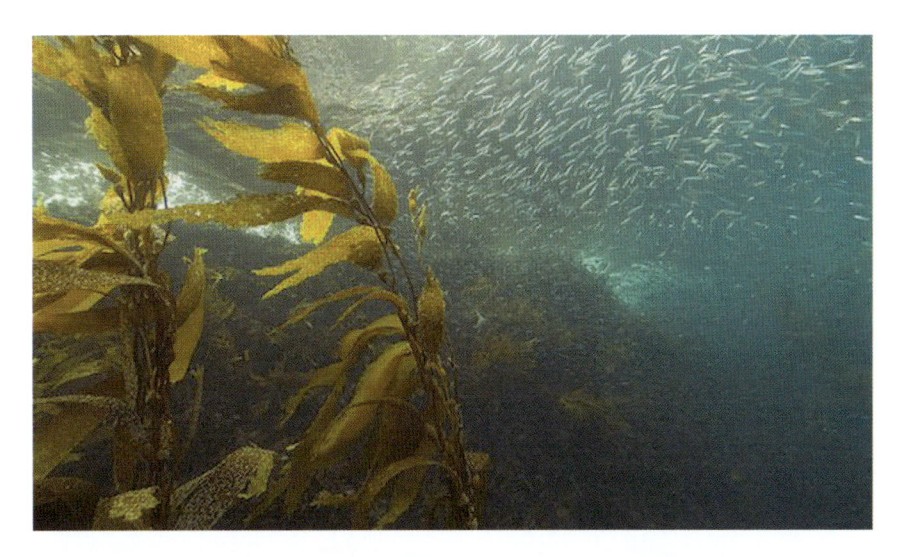

Keywords: disorientated, unification, calm, empower, synchronisation, dizziness, imbalances, before and after travel

Indications: working as one. Good for when you are feeling disorientated, after travelling, holidays – going back to school, work etc.

Healing Qualities: After a spiritual retreat experience or intense workshop, course – bringing you back so that you can cope with the 'real' world.

For when one aspect of yourself is too dominant e. g. the body, mind or spirit, and needs to be brought back into alignment with the others so that you can function as a whole and balanced person.

Mull

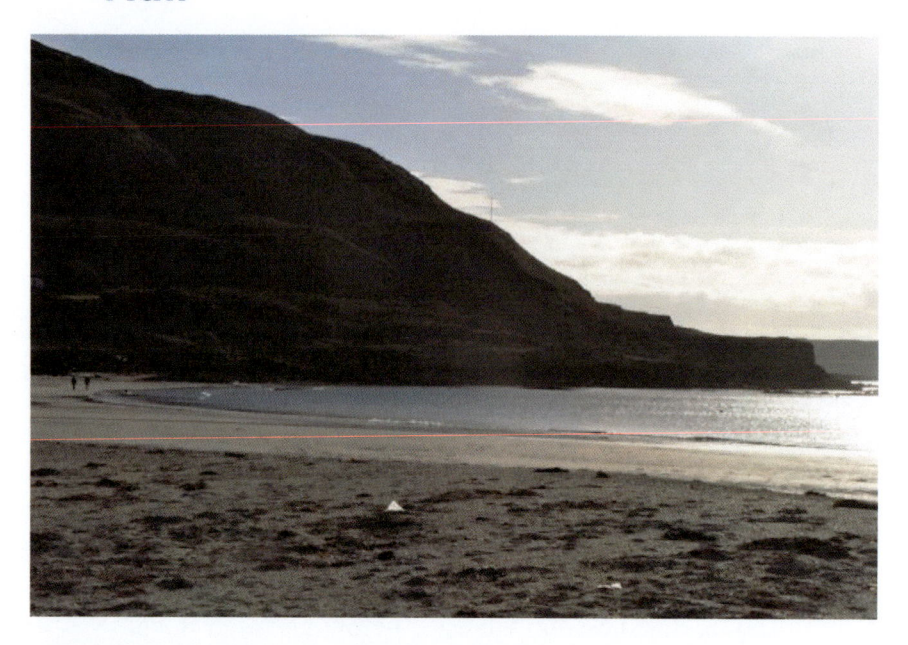

Keywords: isolation, loneliness, forlornness, displaced, bereft, emptiness, depression, turmoil, trauma, melancholia, belonging, land, balance, equilibrium,

Indications: This essence is for isolation, loneliness, forlornness, melancholy It is about wanting to belong. Wanting to be loved. Feelings of being displaced.

It will address these feelings and bring us back to equilibrium.

Healing Qualities: It will settle down the pain within the emotional centres, when we are bereft, empty. Feeling displaced so out of kilter and encountering trauma which is overwhelming, it seems too much to bear. This is an essence that will bring us back to a state of balance.

It is also a really effective on the land bringing bale.

Jan Rose's Insights:
This essence holds the land and its beings within the heart, Land, People, Animals.
Land healing acts as a bridge between earth beings, depleted or unhappy land might not wish to communicate with humans, but by using this essence on the place (remotely if necessary), a connection can be made with strong vibrant beings from an unspoilt and healthy place who can help them directly. A land healing intermediary.

Use in prayer/meditation (group or alone) for the healing of the land. Helps to make a connection with Mull land spirits who can help and give strength to those others who are under attack

Oxwich Bay

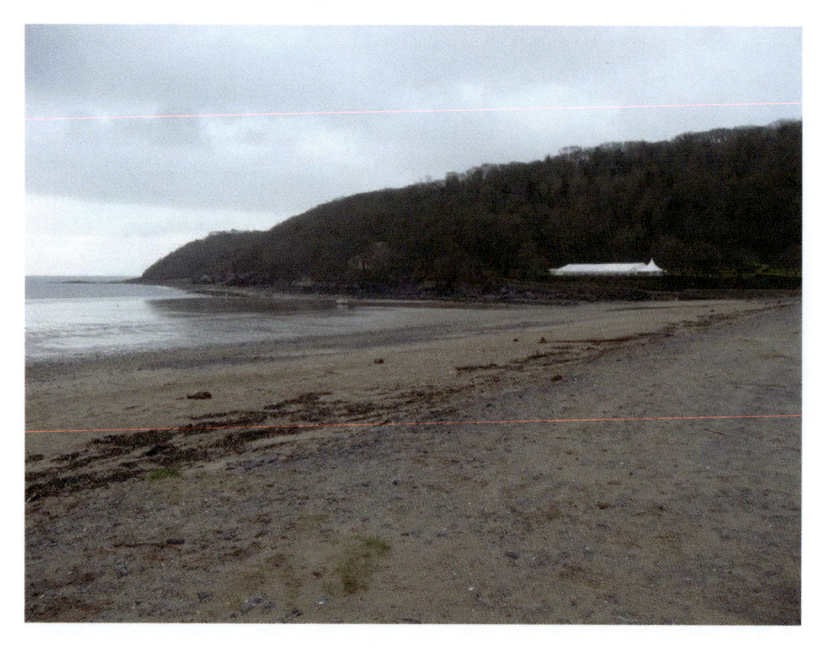

Keywords: intimidate, bullied, abuse, disturbance, non-reactive, tranquillity, clarity, cleanse, cleaner, psychic disturbance, powerful clearer

Indications: Throat chakra, This essence is about being able to step back, out of situations and to remain none reactive. Helps us to take a view on situations and bring clarity and tranquillity.
useful for people who are being bullied or intimidated, at work, at school, at home, etc

Shuts down bad psychic energy very effectively and quickly. Its like having a tonic, taking a pick me up.

Healing Qualities: This has been an essence that has been used with victims of domestic abuse, also for people subjected to bullying, helping us to step back and not react.
It will Keep working, until original energy is broken-down and reduced, cleansed and brought into another better cleaner, clearer form. Cleansing, reducing and reworking an energy problem,

relentlessly pounding it into shape with repetitive rhythmical movements.

It could be a useful essence to use alongside drumming, rattling on oppressive or aggressive energies, This is very effective in cleansing places or object particularly if linked into and being used in an unethical manner. It will deal very quickly and effectively.

Very effective for psychic attack, helps if you visualise waves crashing down on the shore and utilise the power.
when I made this essence I had been going through a difficult time and was on retreat. I collected several different seaweeds. I made this essence in the garden overlooking the bay. And this powerful essence was the result.
Upon my return I was able to stand back and not be so reactive, to the situation.

this has come up on a few occasions where people are in a situation where they are being bullied. One woman was being physically abused, it certainly seemed to help her step back and be less reactive.

Notes: *Jan Rose's Insights:*
Can feel tide in my hand, sea crashing powerfully onto rocks into pebbles, breaking them down and smoothing them into lesser jagged forms. Further pounding them down into grains of sand. On and on relentlessly. The breaking down of adverse energies or problems.

Runswick-Bay

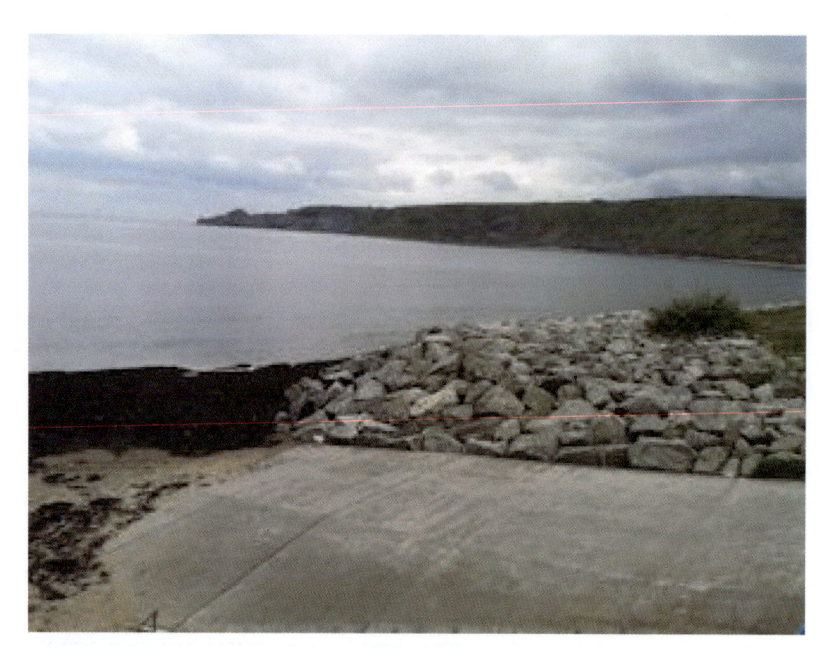

Keywords: balance, rebalances

Indications: 3eye, ears, when you are struggling with keeping or finding the balance

Healing Qualities: this essence is all about finding balance. It often comes up for clients who struggle to find balance in life.

Notes: Made this one day when I went up to Runswick Bay for the day. As I was pouring the essence into the jug I was struggling to find the balance. Then to my amusement I watched as people clamber over rocks and keeping their balance. I just love the way essences work and the way spirit teaches us.

Sea Lettuce

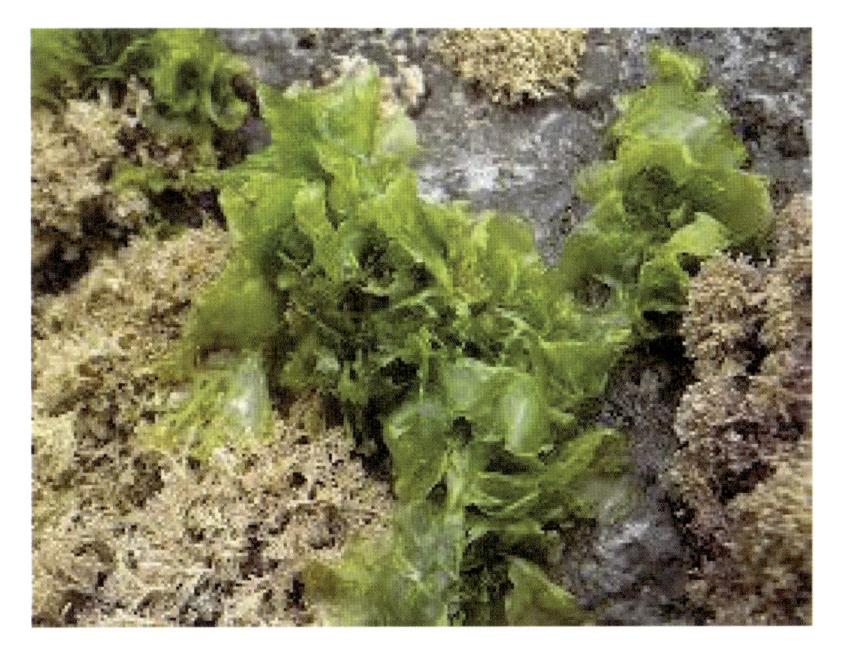

Keywords: tension, undercurrents, enables, smooths, flow

Indications: Heart chakra, ebb and flow. This essence works with the currents, it smooths things out.

Healing Qualities: Because this essence works with the currents within situations, it will help things to flow properly.
We may be dealing with tensions but don't know what they are, but can feel those undercurrents. It will help bring those difficulties to the surface enabling things to run less intensely.

Ulva

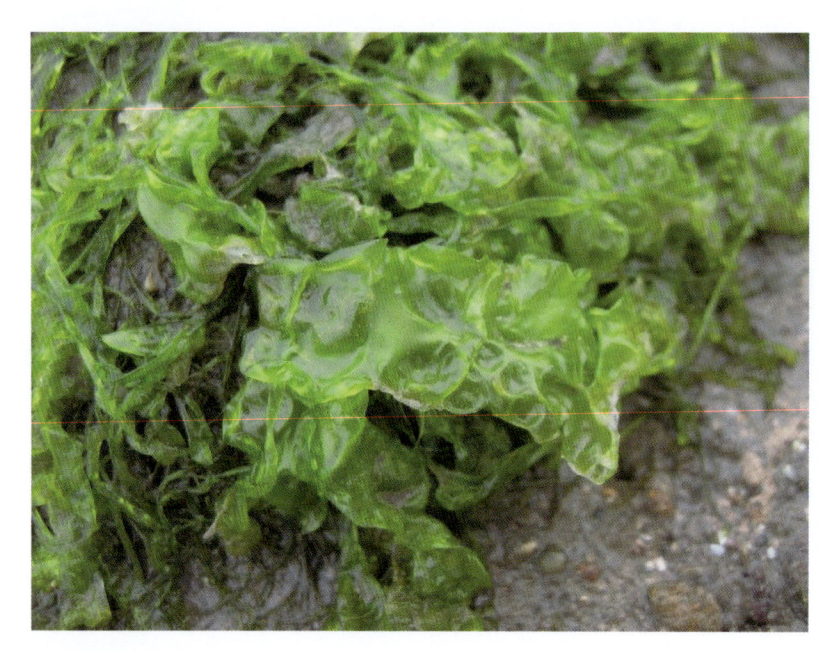

Keywords: cleaning, cleanses, refreshing, declutter, letting go, release, invigorates, chi-balancer,

Indications: Throat chakra,
Could be useful for releasing anything that no longer serves us and needs to go, whether that is emotionally, or psychically.
Could be really useful when moving house and we are needing to declutter.

Healing Qualities: Taking away that which is no longer needed but which we feel we cannot release; removing it and breaking it down into manageable small particles. Helpful for when we need to declutter our lives on all levels. Helps us to feel the exhilaration of truly letting go.

That which has felt immense and important and immovable can now be seen for what it truly is.

Notes: *Jan Rose's insights*
Can hear the tides again, but stronger and much more forceful than with the Seaweed Kelp.
Tides crashing vigorously onto the shingled beach, pushing up to the shore, then pulling debris away back into the ocean with them.

White-Bay

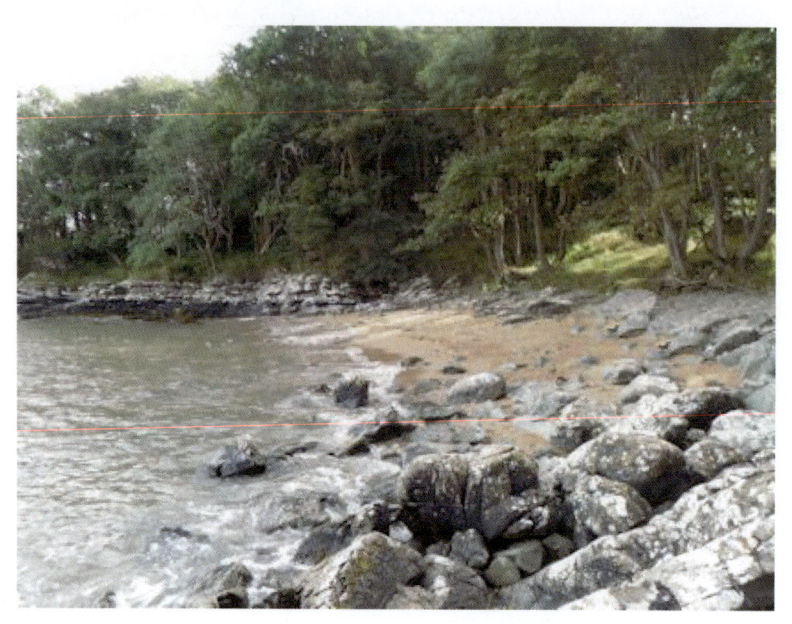

Keywords: reconciliation, clarity, self-aware,

Indications: reconciliation within oneself.

Healing Qualities: during the time this essence was being birthed from several sea weeds in a place called White Bay, I found myself putting to rights things that I had been in conflict. Reflecting on friendships, family, situations. Also, it has come in useful for clients and helps them to come to terms with things that have or are dealing with.

Helen ward often back up the information that has already presented itself.
clarity of self, you do what suits you, you make your own rules and work in the best way for you, which will naturally, be the best for the ones you care for. reconciliation is part of this.

this essence helps one find ones journey through life, perhaps how to walk through life in the way one needs to. We are all putting on the show of our lives!

Seaweed Combination

For earth & water healing – not to be taken orally

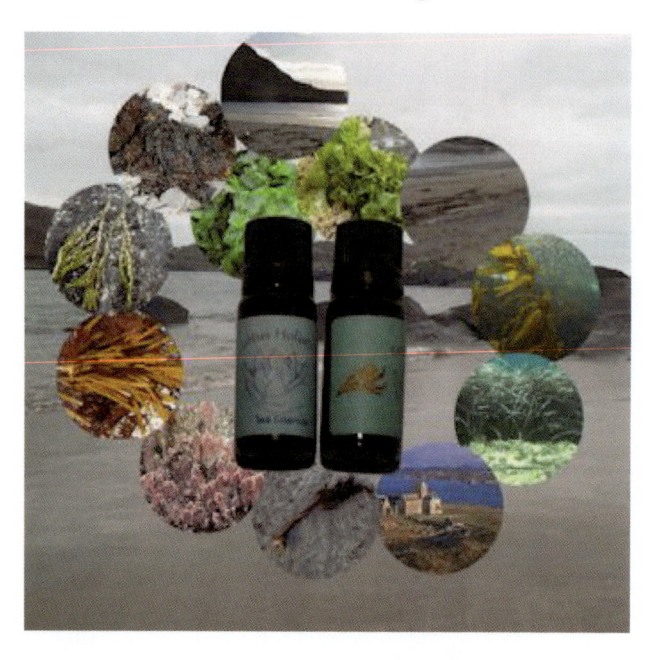

Keywords: ceremony, ritual, honouring, clears, protection, harmonisation, ley lines, closing portals, energetic disturbances,

Indications: This essence only gets used for ceremony on land and water.
it is an effective land and water clearer.

Healing Qualities: This is a combination of all the seaweed mixed together and Pearl is included. it is a very powerful mix. Taken Orally it is totally life changing and will affect the transformation and growth necessary to return to your intended path in life. It is an essence that you would brace yourself! It certainly comes into its own when used in ceremony and ritual work It is a really effective on land and water clearer.
People are working with it all over the world either by participation in groups or as individuals for re-connecting disturbed ley lines,

closing portals etc. For Example; it has been used by anti-fracking groups and on old bomb sites with interesting effects. At a disturbed level it will help balance any disturbed or disturbing energies in your house and garden to effect peace and harmony.

used with anti fracking groups it has had some very interesting effects.

at a simpler level it will help balance any disturbing energies in your house and garden to effect peace and harmony

Combination Essences

Back-On-Track

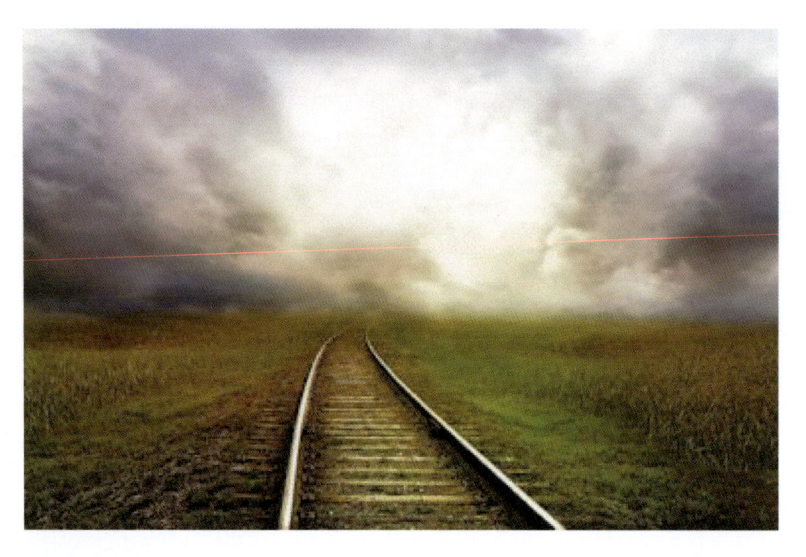

Keywords: direction, focus, anchor, realigns, discombobulated, turmoil

Indications: when life events has blown you off course, it gets you 'Back on track'.

Healing Qualities: in our current times of crisis when facing the immense challenges, which have thrown us into complete disarray, we have become totally disorientated . This combination realigns and gets you 'Back on Track'.

Chillax

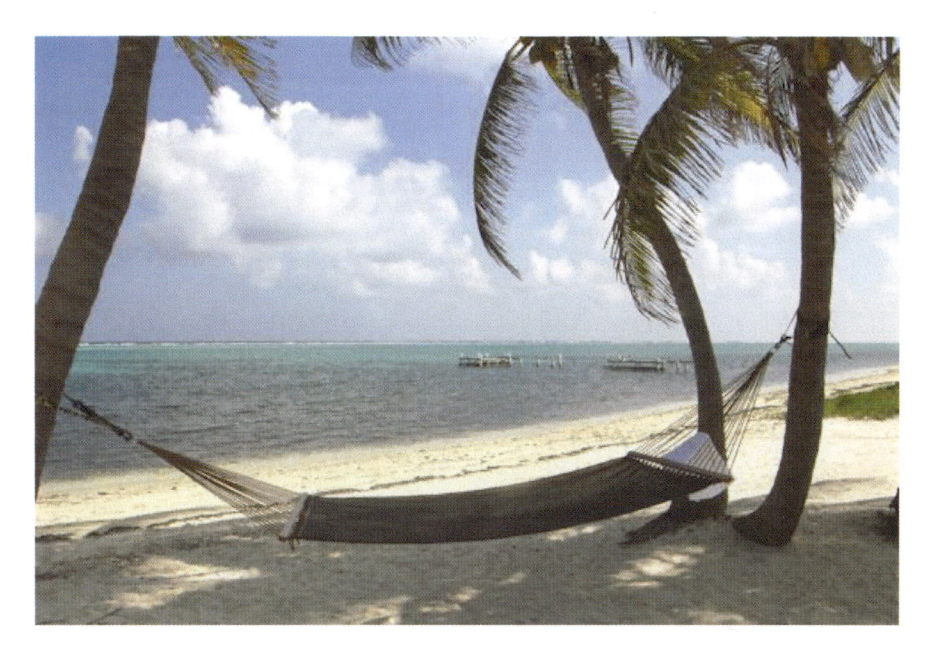

Keywords: relax, calm, emotions, slumber,

Indications: This combination of essences helps to unwind, breaking free of restraints and limitations. Will help us at the end of the day as we enter the dark hours to relax and rest.

Healing Qualities: Helps to refresh and give deep relaxation. Refreshing our whole state of being.

Constellation Mix

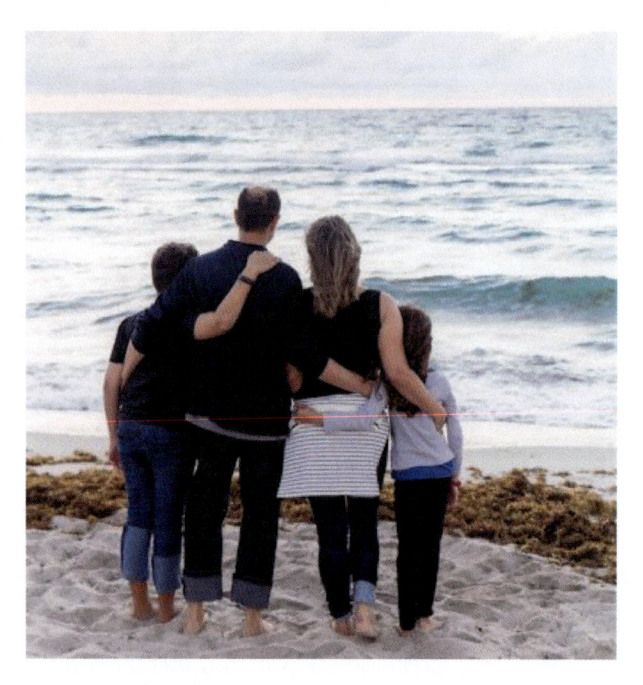

Keywords: DNA, ancestral, disturbance, ancestral, strength, supports

Indications: When ancestral work is being done, this helps settle the DNA and reduce disturbance.
This essence supports working with the ancestors.

Healing Qualities: This essence helps the effects of the work to settle things down. Helping to accept the outcome.

Electro Protector

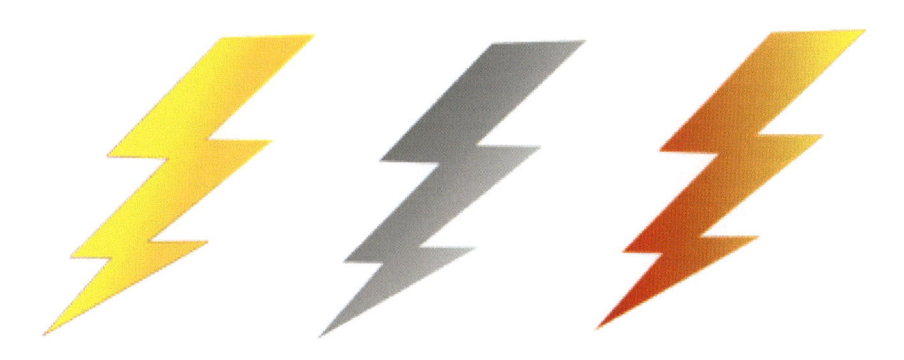

Keywords: computers, settles, energy

Indications: Leave an unopened bottle by your computer or electronic equipment to settle the energies.
Can be made into a spray and used around computers and to clear the energies that is created.

Exam Study

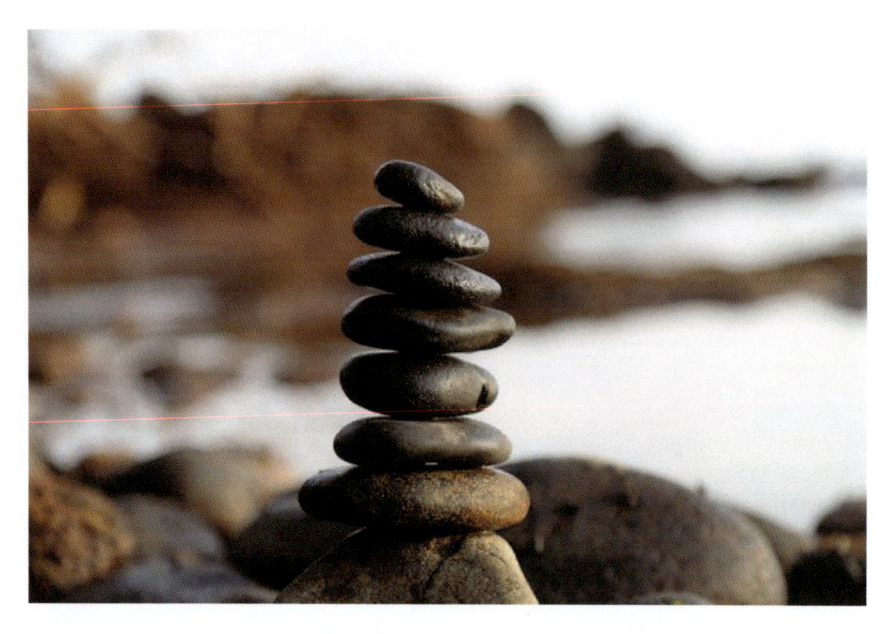

Keywords: nerves, anxiety, fear, focus, exam, memory, new skills

Indications: Anxiety, Nerves, Fear, Ambition all play a part in the success of the candidate for an exam.

Healing Qualities: This essence will help soothe the path, and help the student recognise all that he or she knows on the subject and be clearer. It will settle you down and help to focus.

Helping Hands

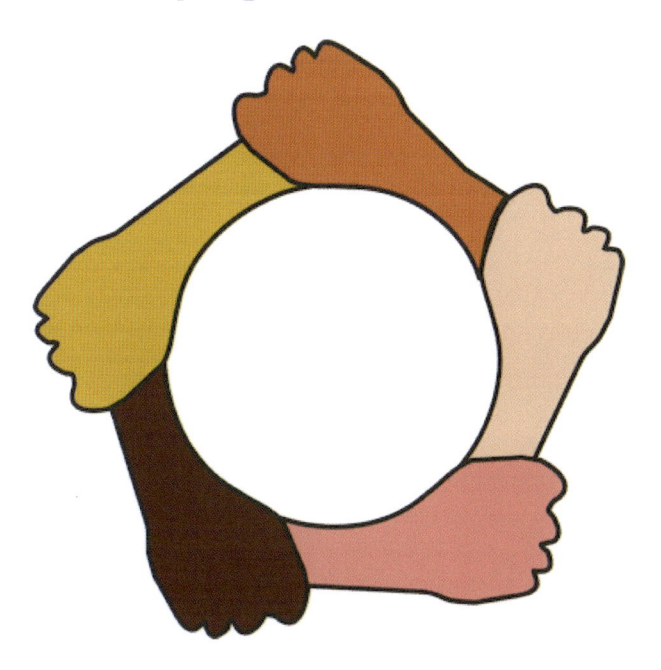

Keywords: balances chakra system, shock, distress, anxiety, focus, alignment, boundaries, stress, emotions, rawness, anchor, emergency, trauma, disorientated,

Indications: Helping Hands is a combination of 5 essences, To gain deeper insights and knowledge into the individual essences refer to the information provided,

Healing Qualities: This is an excellent combination, which helps when challenges take us to the brink, leaving us feeling out of kilter and totally disorientated, helping with focus. When there is high stress, helps to anchor.
People who use this combination find it really useful when stress and anxiety have destabilised the emotions. It realigns us back into ourselves and helps to re-focus.

Notes: Helping-Hands is a combination of 5 essences

Christmas-Cacti-Sun,
Rhododendron,
Kerria Japonica,
White Rambling Rose,
Inipi Moss

Recuperation

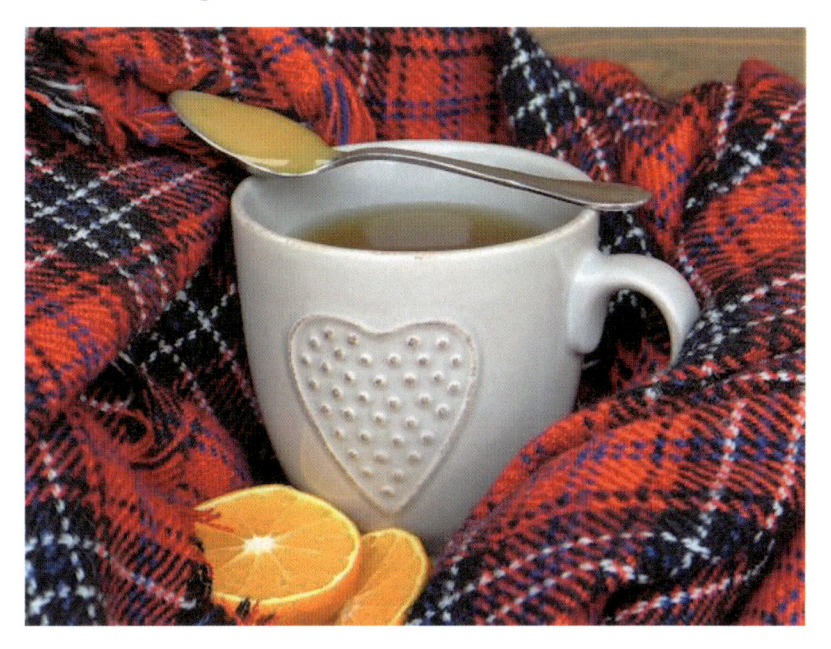

Keywords: Recuperation, perspective, perception, insight, soul insight, strength, recover, receptivity, concentration,

Indications: it strengthens our resolve, particularly when we are recovering from disorders that we encounter. An essence for the soul, it reminds us at a deep level of our DNA/design that needs to be switched on or reminding us of it. It connects into the language of light.

Healing Qualities: Recuperation is to remind the suffering soul on earth how to re-connect with life and mission, to remind us of our special purpose, what ever is being recovered from part of it is to recover some of the key things.

This combination was created for people who were dealing with the ill effects during illness or long term can aid with balancing our bodies. Helps to support with changes in our perception of ourselves, bringing insights which previously we weren't aware of, dealing with the challenge of what has ailed us. When we emerge from these trials we often have a different perspective, these insights we may gain glimpses of what our souls future is about.

Notes: I was guided when two people contacted me suffering from Covid and the same combination came up for both. This combination has also come up for others. When looking at the combination it made total sense.

Sunshine Lift

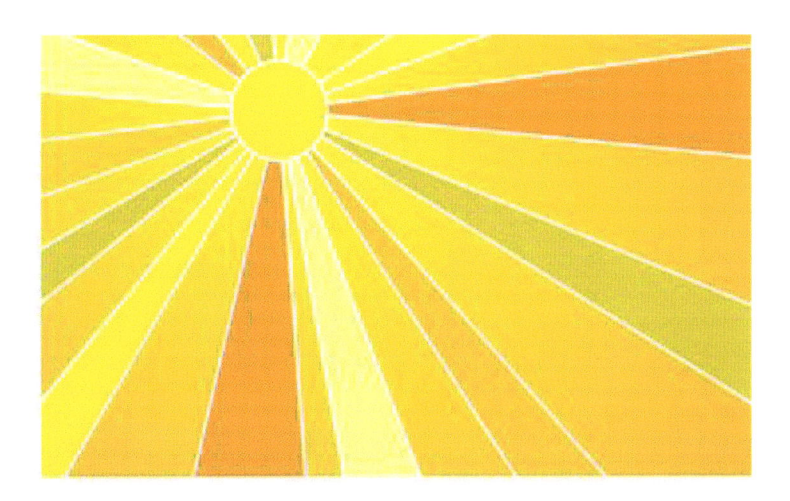

Keywords: depression, SAD, melancholia, uplifts, weary, grief,

Indications: depression, SAD, it can help lift the spirit.

Healing Qualities: This combination essence helps with depression, those who struggle with SAD supporting through the dark days in our lives. Lifting the spirit. From mild, dark cloud descending, to depression that is affecting us on a day to day basis, when we are dealing with grief. Helps us find the strength to carry on. Brings the sunshine back into our lives., the' joie de vivre'

Alphabetical List of All Essences

Angelica seed
Apple Blossom
Back-On-Track
Basalt
Belladonna
Bifurcaria
Black Cohosh
Black-Eyed-Susan (Rudbeckia)
Blackpool Mill
Blackthorn
Bluebell
Boneset-Eupatorium-Perfoliatum
Borage
Bridging-the-Gap
Buddleia
Caherdaniel Bladderwrack
Calendula
Camellia
Castor Oil Plant
Chamomile
Cherry Blossom
Chicory
Chillax
Christmas Cacti (Moon)
Christmas Cacti (Sun)
Christmas Rose (cream)
Clary-sage
Constellation Mix
Corallejo - Halimeda tuna
Coralline
Cornflower
Cowslip
Cranesbill
Creeping Buttercup
Derrynane Kelp
Echinacea
Elderflower
Electro Protector
Exam Study
Forget me Not
Forsythia
Foxglove (pink)
Galactic-Configuration
Gingko-Biloba
Great-Burnet
Hazel Catkin
Helping Hands
Henbane
Hibiscus
Holly
Honesty
Inipi Moss

Iona
Iris-Germanic
Ivy
Japanese Azalea
Japanese Azalea (Saki)
Kefalonia
Kefalonia Bamboo
Kelp
Kelp-holdfast
Kerria Japonica
Lacy-Phacelia
Ladies Mantle
Lambs Ears
Laurel
Lavender
Lotus
Mahonia
Mandrake
Marsh-Mallow
Medlar
Mimulus
Money Plant
Montbretia
Mull
Mullein
Nettle
New Zealand Flax
Obsidian
Orange Blossom
Ox Eye Daisy

Oxwich Bay
Peace Lily
Pear
Pearl
Peony
Pink Dog Rose
Pink/White Hawthorn
Plum
Poke root
Pomegranate
Pulsatilla
Rainbow-Warrior
Recuperation
Red Flowering Currant
Rhododendron
Rhubarb
Rosebay Willowherb
Rosemary
Rowan Berry
Rowan Blossom
Runswick-Bay
Scabious
Scotch-Thistle
Scurvy-Grass
Sea Lettuce
Seaweed
Self Heal
Snow Drop
St-Johns-Wort
Sunshine Lift

Sycamore
Tobacco
Torbay Palm
Turkey-Tail-Bracket-Fungus
Turkish-Filbert
Ulva
Valerian
Viburnum Burkwoodii
Vipers-Bugloss
White Dog Rose
White Hawthorn
White Lilac
White Rambling Rose
White Sage
White Spirea
White-Bay
Wild Garlic
Willow
Wisteria
Yarrow
Yellow-Poppy

Index of Keywords

abundance
    Christmas Rose (cream) 39
    Money Plant 81
abuse
    Black Cohosh 145
    Oxwich Bay 218
acceptance
    Bluebell 28
    Elderflower 45
    Scurvy-Grass 181
access
    Forget me Not 47
achieving
    Basalt 189
action
    Kerria Japonica 66
activator
    Mandrake 76
adapt
    Elderflower 45
adaptability
    Clary-sage 159
    Torbay Palm 121
addictions
    Apple Blossom 26
    Buddleia 30
    Forsythia 49
    Kelp 214
    Lacy-Phacelia 170
    Ladies Mantle 68
    Tobacco 183
adjust
    Orange Blossom 88
adoption
    Torbay Palm 121
adversity
    Plum 101
aggression
    Holly 56
    Pink/White Hawthorn 99
agitation
    Torbay Palm 121
aims
    Cornflower 41
Akashic records
    Bifurcaria 201
    Viburnum Burkwoodii 124
alert
    Rosebay Willowherb 110
alignment
    Helping Hands 233
    Money Plant 81
aligns
    Bifurcaria 201
all chakra's
    Rowan Berry 112
aloofness
    Iona 211
ancestral
    Apple Blossom 26
    Buddleia 30
    Chamomile 157
    Constellation Mix 230
    Elderflower 45
    Forsythia 49
    Gingko-Biloba 52
    Henbane 165
    Mahonia 74
    Pink/White Hawthorn 99
    Torbay Palm 121
anchor
    Back-On-Track 228
    Christmas Cacti (Sun) 37
    Galactic-Configuration 197
    Helping Hands 233
    Mandrake 76
    Poke root 175
    Pomegranate 102
    Rowan Berry 112
    St-Johns-Wort 182
    Torbay Palm 121
angelic
    Cherry Blossom 34
anger
    Chamomile 156
    Derrynane Kelp 210

Holly 56
Mahonia 74
Marsh-Mallow 173
Nettle 85
Poke root 175
animal
    Kelp 214
anorexia
    Belladonna 143
anxiety
    Exam Study 232
    Helping Hands 233
    Marsh-Mallow 173
    Mimulus 79
    Rhubarb 108
    Scotch-Thistle 180
    St-Johns-Wort 182
aspirations
    Cornflower 41
assertive
    Cranesbill 43
attachments
    Black Cohosh 145
aura 43
    Cranesbill 43
    White Sage 133
authentic
    Bluebell 28
    Lavender 172
    Orange Blossom 88
    Rainbow-Warrior 199
awareness
    Cornflower 41
    Rosebay Willowherb 110
balance
    Basalt 189
    Black Cohosh 145
    Inipi Moss 59
    Mull 216
    Poke root 175
    Rosemary 179
    Runswick-Bay 220
    Self Heal 115
balances
    Blackthorn 149
    Japanese Azalea (Saki) 63
    Money Plant 81
    Pink Dog Rose 98
balances chakra system
    Helping Hands 233
balances chakras
    White Spirea 134
battered
    Japanese Azalea 61
    Montbretia 83
beauty
    Scurvy-Grass 181
before and after travel
    Kelp-holdfast 215
belonging
    Mull 216
bereft
    Mull 216
birth
    Apple Blossom 26
    Black Cohosh 145
blockages
    Torbay Palm 121
blocked
    Iris-Germanic 167
    Lavender 172
boundaries
    Helping Hands 233
    Iris-Germanic 167
    Mandrake 76
    Red Flowering Currant 104
    Rhododendron 106
breaking patterns
    Chamomile 157
breath
    Lacy-Phacelia 170
brightness of spirit
    Medlar 78
bruised by life
    Japanese Azalea 61
Bruised/battered by life
    Mullein 174
bullied
    Oxwich Bay 218
burdened
    Blackthorn 149
    Cowslip 160
burn out
    Black-Eyed-Susan 147

calm
  Chillax 229
  Iona 211
  Kelp-holdfast 215
calmness
  Clary-sage 159
  Money Plant 81
calms
  Blackthorn 149
  Caherdaniel Bladderwrack 206
  Great-Burnet 163
  Hibiscus 55
  Scotch-Thistle 180
calms inner turmoil
  Marsh-Mallow 173
cares hope
  Red Flowering Currant 104
centring
  Cranesbill.. 43
ceremony
  Seaweed Combination 226
chakras
  Angelica seed 141
  Coralline 208
  Lambs Ears 69
  Peace Lily 93
  Yarrow... 186
challenges
  Torbay Palm 121
change
  Bluebell 28
  Kelp 214
chaos
  Caherdaniel Bladderwrack 206
  Calendula 154
  Clary-sage 159
  Galactic-Configuration 197
  Pomegranate................................... 102
  White Lilac....................................... 128
cheerfulness
  Torbay Palm 121
chi
  Hibiscus 55
chi-balancer
  Ulva 222
child-like
  Turkish-Filbert 123

chillax
  Chamomile 156
clarifies
  Coralline 208
  Mandrake 76
  Ox Eye Daisy 91
clarity
  Basalt... 189
  Belladonna....................................... 143
  Bifurcaria 201
  Chamomile 157
  Foxglove (pink) 51
  Gingko-Biloba 52
  Ivy.. 168
  Japanese Azalea 61
  Japanese Azalea (Saki)................... 63
  Lotus 72
  Oxwich Bay 218
  Rosemary.. 179
  Scabious 114
  Self Heal.. 115
  White Hawthorn.............................. 127
  White-Bay... 224
  Willow 137
Clarity
  Angelica seed.................................. 141
cleaner
  Oxwich Bay 218
cleaning
  Ulva 222
cleanse
  Ladies Mantle 68
  Montbretia 83
  Oxwich Bay 218
  White Sage 133
cleanser
  Blackpool Mill 204
  Red Flowering Currant................... 104
cleanses
  Kefalonia.. 213
  Kefalonia Bamboo 65
  Ulva 222
  White Lilac....................................... 128
  Wild Garlic 136
cleansing
  Black Cohosh 145
clears

Blackthorn 149
   Seaweed Combination 226
   White Lilac 128
   Wild Garlic 136
closing portals
   Seaweed Combination 226
clutter
   Ox Eye Daisy 91
   Poke root 175
co-dependency
   Tobacco 183
comfort
   Snow Drop 117
commotion
   Elderflower 45
communication
   Vipers-Bugloss 185
Community
   Borage 152
compassion 56
   Holly 56
   Peony 96
completion
   Pearl 193
complicated
   White Dog Rose 126
computers
   Electro Protector 231
concealed
   Forget me Not 47
concentration
   Recuperation 235
conditioning
   Chamomile 157
confidence
   Buddleia 30
   Camellia 31
   Cranesbill 43
   Hazel Catkin 54
   Laurel 70
   Mimulus 79
   Montbretia 83
   Rhubarb 108
   Rosebay Willowherb 110
   Rowan Berry 112
conflict
   Bifurcaria 201
   Chamomile 156
   Gingko-Biloba 52
   Great-Burnet 163
   Hazel Catkin 54
   Snow Drop 117
conflicts
   Nettle 85
confusion
   Bifurcaria 201
   Foxglove (pink) 51
   Hazel Catkin 54
   Rosebay Willowherb 110
   White Lilac 128
congested energy
   Castor Oil Plant 33
congestion
   Scabious 114
connection
   Christmas Cacti (Sun) 37
   Christmas Rose (cream) 39
   Rosebay Willowherb 110
connections
   Ivy 168
   Nettle 85
connects
   Christmas Cacti (Moon) 35
consolidation
   Basalt 189
constraint
   Christmas Cacti (Moon) 35
control
   Great-Burnet 163
convalescing
   Lacy-Phacelia 170
core strength
   Rhododendron 106
   Rowan Berry 112
courage
   Black Cohosh 145
   Christmas Cacti (Moon) 35
   Forsythia 49
   Mahonia 74
   Mandrake 76
   Scotch-Thistle 180
   Self Heal 115
creativity
   Iris-Germanic 167

crisis
  Scotch-Thistle 180
crone
  Black Cohosh 145
Cross-roads
  Henbane 165
curses
  Henbane 165
cushions
  White Rambling Rose 131
custody battles
  Pink/White Hawthorn 99
dark night of soul
  Iona 211
death
  Henbane 165
deceptions
  Ivy 168
decision
  Hazel Catkin 54
  White Hawthorn 127
decisions
  Montbretia 83
decisive
  Angelica seed 141
declutter
  Ulva 222
de-clutter
  Blackpool Mill 204
deep melancholia
  Iona 211
deep sadness
  Calendula 154
  Creeping Buttercup 44
  Forsythia 49
  Wisteria 138
deep trauma
  Echinacea 161
defences
  Peony 96
deflection
  Obsidian 191
delight
  Turkish-Filbert 123
depleted
  Boneset 150
depressed

Lavender 172
depression
  Buddleia 30
  Calendula 154
  Creeping Buttercup 44
  Iona 211
  Mull 216
  St-Johns-Wort 182
  Sunshine Lift 237
desolation
  Forsythia 49
despair
  Blackthorn 149
  Iris-Germanic 167
destiny
  Rainbow-Warrior 199
detachment
  Obsidian 191
determination
  Scabious 114
diminish
  Rowan Berry 112
direction
  Back-On-Track 228
  Forsythia 49
  Viburnum Burkwoodii 124
discernment
  Iona 211
  White Hawthorn 127
discipline
  Mahonia 74
discombobulated
  Back-On-Track 228
  Lavender 172
disconnected
  Ivy 168
  Valerian 184
disconnection
  Iona 211
  Rosebay Willowherb 110
disgruntled
  Iris-Germanic 167
dismal
  Cherry Blossom 34
disorientated
  Helping Hands 233
  Kelp-holdfast 215

displaced
  Mull 216
  Torbay Palm 121
distorted view
  Belladonna 143
distress
  Coralline 208
  Helping Hands 233
disturbance
  Constellation Mix 230
  Oxwich Bay 218
divorce
  Pink/White Hawthorn 99
  White Hawthorn 127
dizziness
  Kelp-holdfast 215
DNA
  Constellation Mix 230
downloader
  Japanese Azalea 61
dreams
  Forget me Not 47
  Viburnum Burkwoodii 124
drive
  Kefalonia Bamboo 65
element rebalancer
  Iona 211
embedded
  Wisteria 138
emergency
  Helping Hands 233
emotion
  Torbay Palm 121
emotional
  Gingko-Biloba 52
emotional /energy cleanser
  Turkey-Tail 187
emotional blockages
  Sycamore 119
emotional rawness
  White Rambling Rose 131
emotional states
  Pulsatilla 178
emotions
  Chillax 229
  Helping Hands 233
  Kerria Japonica 66

Sycamore 119
Valerian 184
empathy
  Pink/White Hawthorn 99
empower
  Coralline 208
  Honesty 58
  Kelp-holdfast 215
  Ladies Mantle 68
empowers
  Rhododendron 106
emptiness
  Mull 216
enables
  Sea Lettuce 221
energetic disturbances
  Seaweed Combination 226
energiser
  Inipi Moss 59
energises
  Black Cohosh 145
energy
  Christmas Cacti (Sun) 37
  Corallejo - Halimeda 207
  Electro Protector 231
  Hibiscus 55
  Japanese Azalea 61
  Kerria Japonica 66
  Money Plant 81
  Ox Eye Daisy 91
energy protection
  Derrynane Kelp 210
environment
  Corallejo - Halimeda 207
envy
  Tobacco 183
equilibrium
  Mull 216
  Pulsatilla 178
estranged family
  Pink/White Hawthorn 99
exam
  Exam Study 232
exhaustion
  Boneset 150
expansive
  Lotus 72

express
    Mandrake 76
faith
    Kelp 214
    Self Heal 115
fatigue
    Blackthorn 149
fear
    Black Cohosh 145
    Bluebell 28
    Borage 152
    Caherdaniel Bladderwrack 206
    Elderflower 45
    Exam Study 232
    Forsythia 49
    Holly 56
    Mahonia 74
    Mimulus 79
    Montbretia 83
    Rhubarb 108
    Scotch-Thistle 180
    St-Johns-Wort 182
    Sycamore 119
feed the spirit
    Buddleia 30
feeling
    Basalt 189
feminine
    Red Flowering Currant 104
feminine power
    Pearl 193
fester
    Blackthorn 149
filters
    Inipi Moss 59
filters emotions
    Kefalonia 213
fire balancer
    Inipi Moss 59
flexibility
    Elderflower 45
    Rhubarb 108
    Tobacco 183
    White Rambling Rose 131
    Willow 137
flow
    Coralline 208
    Lotus 72
    Sea Lettuce 221
flustered
    Bluebell 28
focus
    Apple Blossom 26
    Back-On-Track 228
    Basalt 189
    Castor Oil Plant 33
    Chamomile 156
    Christmas Cacti (Sun) 37
    Cornflower 41
    Exam Study 232
    Forget me Not 47
    Hazel Catkin 54
    Helping Hands 233
    Kelp 214
    Lambs Ears 69
    White Spirea 134
forgiveness
    New Zealand Flax 86
    Orange Blossom 88
    Peace Lily 93
forlornness
    Mull 216
fortitude
    Mahonia 74
    Obsidian 191
fragile 131
Fragile
    Yellow-Poppy 140
frazzled
    Pomegranate 102
frazzled mind
    Lavender 172
freedom
    Hazel Catkin 54
    Japanese Azalea 61
frustration
    Iris-Germanic 167
fulfilment
    Torbay Palm 121
gateway
    Willow 137
generational
    Chamomile 157
generosity

Pink Dog Rose 98
gentleness
　　Peony 96
geopathic stress
　　Peace Lily 93
gloomy
　　Cherry Blossom 34
　　Self Heal 115
go with the flow
　　Bluebell 28
good will
　　Cherry Blossom 34
gratitude
　　Christmas Rose (cream) 39
　　Self Heal 115
gratitude rebirth
　　Mullein 174
grief
　　Borage 152
　　Pear 95
　　Snow Drop 117
　　Sunshine Lift 237
　　Wisteria 138
grounding
　　Basalt 189
　　Christmas Cacti (Sun) 37
　　Inipi Moss 59
　　Ivy 168
　　Mandrake 76
　　Poke root 175
　　Rhododendron 106
　　Rosebay Willowherb 110
　　Rowan Berry 112
　　Tobacco 183
grounds
　　Galactic-Configuration 197
　　Scotch-Thistle 180
　　Viburnum Burkwoodii 124
growth
　　Rhododendron 106
grumpy
　　Cherry Blossom 34
guidance
　　Pomegranate 102
gut-feeling
　　Honesty 58
habit breakers

　　Apple Blossom 26
habits
　　Apple Blossom 26
happiness
　　Calendula 154
　　Cherry Blossom 34
hard hearted
　　Marsh-Mallow 173
harmonisation
　　Christmas Cacti (Sun) 37
　　Money Plant 81
　　Seaweed Combination 226
harmonises
　　Gingko-Biloba 52
harmony
　　Holly 56
harness
　　Kerria Japonica 66
head overloaded
　　Rowan Berry 112
healer
　　Pulsatilla 178
healing
　　Angelica seed 141
　　Pink/White Hawthorn 99
health
　　Self Heal 115
healthy
　　Ivy 168
heart
　　Bluebell 28
　　Camellia 31
　　Cowslip 160
　　Foxglove (pink) 51
　　Great-Burnet 163
　　Holly 56
　　Pink/White Hawthorn 99
heart chakra
　　Cranesbill 43
　　Pulsatilla 178
heart warming
　　Pink/White Hawthorn 99
heart-break
　　Camellia 31
　　Snow Drop 117
heavy hearted
　　Cowslip 160

Helping Hands
　　Christmas Cacti (Sun) 37
hidden
　　Forget me Not 47
hidden knowledge
　　Viburnum Burkwoodii 124
higher perspective
　　White Spirea 134
hold space
　　Gingko-Biloba 52
hold steady
　　Galactic-Configuration 197
holding
　　Christmas Rose (cream) 39
home
　　Rainbow-Warrior 199
homesick
　　Torbay Palm 121
honesty
　　Honesty 58
honouring
　　Seaweed Combination 226
hope
　　Blackthorn 149
　　Snow Drop 117
　　White Hawthorn 127
hope lost
　　Self Heal 115
humility
　　Cornflower 41
humour
　　Medlar 78
Identification
　　Borage 152
identity
　　Cowslip 160
　　Echinacea 161
　　Viburnum Burkwoodii 124
illusion
　　Henbane 165
imbalances
　　Kelp-holdfast 215
impartial
　　White Hawthorn 127
incapacitates
　　Lacy-Phacelia 170
indecision

Mullein 174
inner guidance
　　Angelica seed 141
　　Clary-sage 159
inner light
　　Mullein 174
inner peace
　　Rosemary 179
inner resources
　　Black-Eyed-Susan 147
inner self
　　Angelica seed 141
　　Mullein 174
inner strength
　　Self Heal 115
inner tranquillity
　　Pomegranate 102
inner-child
　　Turkey-Tail 187
insight
　　Lotus 72
　　Recuperation 235
　　Self Heal 115
insights
　　Forget me Not 47
　　Inipi Moss 59
integrates
　　Pear 95
integrity
　　Echinacea 161
interdimensional
　　Gingko-Biloba 52
interfere
　　Medlar 78
interference
　　Medlar 78
intimidate
　　Mahonia 74
　　Oxwich Bay 218
intimidated
　　Mahonia 74
invigorates
　　Iona 211
　　Ulva 222
irritable
　　Cherry Blossom 34
irritation

Chamomile 156
Derrynane Kelp 210
Holly 56
isolation
Mull 216
jealousy
Holly 56
joy
Apple Blossom 26
Blackthorn 149
Cherry Blossom 34
Christmas Rose (cream) 39
Snow Drop 117
judgement
Rhubarb 108
White Hawthorn 127
kindness
Cornflower 41
Pink Dog Rose 98
labour
Clary-sage 159
land
Corallejo - Halimeda 207
Kelp 214
Montbretia 83
Mull 216
laughter
Calendula 154
letting go
Black Cohosh 145
Chamomile 157
Marsh-Mallow 173
New Zealand Flax 86
Orange Blossom 88
Ulva 222
letting-go
Chamomile 156
ley lines
Seaweed Combination 226
life tensions
Bifurcaria 201
lifts
Buddleia 30
lifts mood
Rosebay Willowherb 110
light
Castor Oil Plant 33

White Hawthorn 127
lightens mood
Chamomile 156
lightness
Cherry Blossom 34
limitations
Christmas Cacti (Moon) 35
loneliness
Borage 152
Mull 216
lonely
Iona 211
loss
Black Cohosh 145
lost soul
Galactic-Configuration 197
lost soul parts
Pomegranate 102
love
Camellia 31
Holly 56
lungs
Pink Dog Rose 98
male/female balance
Poke root 175
manifesting
Basalt 189
Foxglove (pink) 51
manifests
Christmas Cacti (Sun) 37
Money Plant 81
meddling
Medlar 78
meditation
Christmas Cacti (Moon) 35
meditations
Viburnum Burkwoodii 124
meditative
Holly 56
melancholia
Calendula 154
Creeping Buttercup 44
Iona 211
Mull 216
St-Johns-Wort 182
Sunshine Lift 237
melancholic

Lavender 172
memory
    Exam Study 232
menopause
    Black Cohosh 145
mental anguish
    Iona 211
    Japanese Azalea 61
mental bodies
    Gingko-Biloba 52
mental congestion
    Blackpool Mill 204
meridians
    Boneset 150
mother hen
    Sycamore 119
motherhood
    Black Cohosh 145
motivator
    Apple Blossom 26
mouth
    Calendula 154
move on
    Gingko-Biloba 52
moving on
    Marsh-Mallow 173
narrow minded
    Tobacco 183
negative body-image
    Belladonna 143
negativity
    White Lilac 128
nerves
    Exam Study 232
networker
    Angelica seed 141
new beginnings
    Lacy-Phacelia 170
    White Hawthorn 127
new skills
    Exam Study 232
night terrors
    Laurel 70
nightmares
    St-Johns-Wort 182
non-reactive
    Oxwich Bay 218
nourishment
    Turkish-Filbert 123
nurtured
    Lacy-Phacelia 170
nurtures
    Buddleia 30
nurturing
    Borage 152
    Creeping Buttercup 44
    Red Flowering Currant 104
    Sycamore 119
objectivity
    Bifurcaria 201
obsessive
    Cornflower 41
obstacles
    Ivy 168
old hurts
    Nettle 85
on course
    Bluebell 28
opener
    Pulsatilla 178
openness
    Medlar 78
optimism
    Christmas Rose (cream) 39
    St-Johns-Wort 182
orders
    Calendula 154
overload
    Rowan Berry 112
overwhelm
    Blackpool Mill 204
overwhelmed
    Willow 137
panic
    Rosebay Willowherb 110
    Scotch-Thistle 180
patience 26
    Apple Blossom 26
    Christmas Rose (cream) 39
    Nettle 85
    Pink Dog Rose 98
    White Hawthorn 127
pattern breaker
    Buddleia 30

Forsythia 49
Japanese Azalea 61
Kelp 214
Ladies Mantle 68
Vipers-Bugloss 185

peace
   Bifurcaria 201
   Black Cohosh 145
   Camellia 31
   Christmas Cacti (Moon) 35
   Christmas Rose (cream) 39
   Gingko-Biloba 52
   Lambs Ears 69
   Mahonia 74
   Montbretia 83
   New Zealand Flax 86
   Orange Blossom 88
   Peace Lily 93
   Pear 95
   Rainbow-Warrior 199
   Rowan Blossom 113
   St-Johns-Wort 182
   Wisteria 138

Peace
   Mullein 174

peace of mind
   Great-Burnet 163
   Valerian 184

people
   Kelp 214

perception
   Recuperation 235

perseverance
   Scabious 114

personal power
   Iris-Germanic 167

perspective
   Blackpool Mill 204
   Foxglove (pink) 51
   Henbane 165
   Recuperation 235

place
   Japanese Azalea 61

positive outlook
   Black-Eyed-Susan 147

possessive
   Tobacco 183

power
   Lotus 72
   Mahonia 74
   Pearl 193
   Rhododendron 106
   Rosemary 179
   Rowan Berry 112

powerful clearer
   Oxwich Bay 218

pregnancy
   Black Cohosh 145

pregnancy support
   Christmas Rose (cream) 39

prioritise
   Basalt 189

prioritising
   Cowslip 160

problems solver
   Bifurcaria 201

procrastinate
   Basalt 189
   Elderflower 45

protection
   Angelica seed 141
   Camellia 31
   Cranesbill 43
   Holly 56
   Ladies Mantle 68
   Obsidian 191
   Rowan Berry 112
   Rowan Blossom 113
   Seaweed Combination 226
   Turkish-Filbert 123
   White Lilac 128
   Wild Garlic 136

protective
   Blackthorn 149
   Rosemary 179
   St-Johns-Wort 182
   Turkey-Tail 187
   Yarrow 186

protector
   Pulsatilla 178

psychic abilities
   Basalt 189

psychic attack
   Obsidian 191

psychic connections
　　Angelica seed 141
psychic disturbance
　　Oxwich Bay 218
psychic protection
　　Laurel 70
PTSD
　　Echinacea 161
　　Valerian 184
puberty
　　Black Cohosh 145
purifies
　　Blackthorn 149
　　Kefalonia 213
　　Rowan Blossom 113
　　White Sage 133
purity
　　White Lilac 128
purpose
　　Bluebell 28
　　Kefalonia Bamboo 65
　　Ladies Mantle 68
　　Lambs Ears 69
quiet strength
　　White Hawthorn 127
quietens
　　Lambs Ears 69
　　Mahonia 74
quietens the mind
　　Scabious 114
rage
　　Nettle 85
　　Poke root 175
Raw
　　Valerian 184
rawness
　　Helping Hands 233
　　Torbay Palm 121
　　Wisteria 138
realign
　　Orange Blossom 88
realignment
　　Black Cohosh 145
realigns
　　Back-On-Track 228
　　Christmas Cacti (Sun) 37
　　Mullein 174

New Zealand Flax 86
　　White Spirea 134
reassure
　　Viburnum Burkwoodii ... 124
rebalances
　　Runswick-Bay 220
rebirth
　　Snow Drop 117
re-birth
　　Henbane 165
rebooting
　　Coralline 208
rebuilds
　　Coralline 208
receptivity
　　Recuperation 235
recharge
　　Iona 211
reconciliation
　　White-Bay 224
reconnects
　　Iona 211
recover
　　Recuperation 235
recuperation
　　Lacy-Phacelia 170
Recuperation
　　Recuperation 235
reflect
　　Angelica seed 141
　　Christmas Rose (cream) ... 39
reflects
　　Rowan Blossom 113
refreshing
　　Ulva 222
regenerate
　　Montbretia 83
regenerates
　　Castor Oil Plant 33
regeneration
　　Torbay Palm 121
regroup
　　Bridging-the-Gap 195
　　Gingko-Biloba 52
reintegrates
　　Echinacea 161
reintegration

New Zealand Flax 86
Orange Blossom 88
relationships
   Bifurcaria 201
   Corallejo - Halimeda 207
   Nettle 85
relax
   Chamomile 156
   Chillax 229
relaxation
   Hibiscus 55
release
   Boneset 150
   Gingko-Biloba 52
   Japanese Azalea (Saki) 63
   Kerria Japonica 66
   Montbretia 83
   New Zealand Flax 86
   Orange Blossom 88
   Peace Lily 93
   Peony 96
   Sycamore 119
   Tobacco 183
   Ulva 222
   Wisteria 138
releases
   Medlar 78
remembrance
   Orange Blossom 88
remote viewing
   White Hawthorn 127
renewal
   Apple Blossom 26
renews
   Blackthorn 149
reorientates
   Boneset 150
repressed
   Lavender 172
resentment
   Holly 56
resets
   Boneset 150
   White Hawthorn 127
resilience
   Buddleia 30
   Elderflower 45

Ivy 168
Peace Lily 93
Rhubarb 108
resistance
   Chamomile 157
resistant
   Mandrake 76
   Peony 96
resolution
   Bifurcaria 201
resolutions
   Ivy 168
resources
   Lacy-Phacelia 170
responsibility
   Poke root 175
   Rowan Blossom 113
restoration
   Self Heal 115
restores
   Coralline 208
   Lacy-Phacelia 170
restrictions
   Christmas Cacti (Moon) 35
reveal
   Forget me Not 47
revealer
   Peony 96
reveller
   Forget me Not 47
revenge
   Holly 56
revives
   Self Heal 115
rhythm
   rhythm 59
rhythms
   Ivy 168
rigidness
   Marsh-Mallow 173
ritual
   Seaweed Combination 226
robust
   Rhododendron 106
roots
   Inipi Moss 59
   Ivy 168

Torbay Palm 121
SAD
    Sunshine Lift 237
sadness
    Cowslip 160
    Snow Drop 117
    Valerian 184
safe
    Bluebell 28
    Caherdaniel Bladderwrack 206
    Camellia 31
    Galactic-Configuration 197
    Mimulus 79
    Pomegranate 102
    Wild Garlic 136
scatter
    Kerria Japonica 66
secure
    Scotch-Thistle 180
security
    Poke root 175
seeing clearly
    Basalt 189
self
    Sycamore 119
self destruction
    Ladies Mantle 68
self determination
    Mandrake 76
self doubt
    Hazel Catkin 54
self esteem
    Belladonna 143
self love
    Pink/White Hawthorn 99
self sacrifice
    Montbretia 83
self worth
    Red Flowering Currant 104
self-aware
    White-Bay 224
self-control
    Mahonia 74
    Poke root 175
self-knowledge
    Mahonia 74
self-love

Camellia 31
Creeping Buttercup 44
Holly 56
self-reliance
    Mahonia 74
serenity
    Christmas Cacti (Moon) 35
settles
    Christmas Cacti (Moon) 35
    Christmas Rose (cream) 39
    Clary-sage 159
    Electro Protector 231
    Hibiscus 55
    White Hawthorn 127
settling at night
    Christmas Cacti (Moon) 35
shifts
    Tobacco 183
shock
    Helping Hands 233
    Kelp 214
    Scotch-Thistle 180
    Valerian 184
simplicity
    White Dog Rose 126
sleep
    Chamomile 156
    St-Johns-Wort 182
slumber
    Chamomile 156
    Chillax 229
smooths
    Lambs Ears 69
    Sea Lettuce 221
solar plexus
    Angelica seed 141
soothes
    Money Plant 81
    Snow Drop 117
    Sycamore 119
soothing
    White Rambling Rose 131
sooths
    Caherdaniel Bladderwrack 206
    Christmas Rose (cream) 39
    Great-Burnet 163
soul

Camellia 31
Cranesbill 43
soul insight
   Recuperation 235
soul parts
   Turkey-Tail 187
soul retrieval
   Pearl 193
space
   Blackpool Mill 204
spirit
   Camellia 31
   Mahonia 74
   Pomegranate 102
stabilise
   Mandrake 76
stabilises
   Blackthorn 149
stability
   Henbane 165
steadfastness
   White Hawthorn 127
straight talking
   Mandrake 76
strength
   Angelica seed 141
   Apple Blossom 26
   Black-Eyed-Susan 147
   Constellation Mix 230
   Cowslip 160
   Cranesbill 43
   Elderflower 45
   Kefalonia Bamboo 65
   Lambs Ears 69
   Mahonia 74
   Mandrake 76
   Obsidian 191
   Poke root 175
   Pomegranate 102
   Recuperation 235
   Rhododendron 106
   Scotch-Thistle 180
   Snow Drop 117
   St-Johns-Wort 182
   White Hawthorn 127
Strength
   Yellow-Poppy 140

stress
   Bifurcaria 201
   Chamomile 156
   Coralline 208
   Helping Hands 233
   Pink/White Hawthorn 99
   Rosebay Willowherb 110
strive
   Laurel 70
stuck
   Bridging-the-Gap 195
   Camellia 31
   Chamomile 157
   Medlar 78
   Self Heal 115
   Tobacco 183
success
   Laurel 70
sunshine
   Calendula 154
sunshine lift
   Calendula 154
support
   Cranesbill 43
   Viburnum Burkwoodii 124
supportive
   Blackthorn 149
   Scabious 114
   Turkish-Filbert 123
supports
   Scotch-Thistle 180
suppression
   Cowslip 160
surrendering
   Boneset 150
sweetness
   Sycamore 119
synchronisation
   Kelp-holdfast 215
taking action
   Basalt 189
tenacity
   Apple Blossom 26
   White Hawthorn 127
tension
   Obsidian 191
   Sea Lettuce 221

third eye
  Angelic Seed 141
thoughts
  Kefalonia 213
throat
  Calendula 154
tie cutting
  Red Flowering Currant 104
time out
  Blackpool Mill 204
timid
  Rhubarb 108
torment
  Hazel Catkin 54
toxic
  Blackthorn 149
  Corallejo - Halimeda 207
tranquillity
  Oxwich Bay 218
transformation
  Black Cohosh 145
  Tobacco 183
transitions
  Angelica seed 141
  Bridging-the-Gap 195
  Marsh-Mallow 173
  White Hawthorn 127
Transitions
  Clary-sage 159
trauma
  Helping Hands 233
  Kelp 214
  Lacy-Phacelia 170
  Mull 216
  Pear 95
  Valerian 184
  Yarrow 186
triggers
  Echinacea 161
true Grit
  Black-Eyed-Susan 147
trust
  Camellia 31
truth
  Honesty 58
turmoil
  Back-On-Track 228

  Caherdaniel Bladderwrack 206
  Elderflower 45
  Japanese Azalea 61
  Mull 216
unblocks
  Boneset 150
  Bridging-the-Gap 195
un-complicate
  Ox Eye Daisy 91
undercurrents
  Sea Lettuce 221
understanding
  Holly 56
  Self Heal 115
unemotional
  Lavender 172
unhappy
  Viburnum Burkwoodii 124
unification
  Kelp-holdfast 215
unsavoury
  Pomegranate 102
unsettled
  Bifurcaria 201
unties knots
  Bifurcaria 201
upbeat
  Cherry Blossom 34
upheaval
  Montbretia 83
uplifts
  Cherry Blossom 34
  Creeping Buttercup 44
  Sunshine Lift 237
  Turkish-Filbert 123
  Wild Garlic 136
uptight
  Hibiscus 55
value
  Scurvy-Grass 181
veil lifter
  Turkish-Filbert 123
victim mentality
  Vipers-Bugloss 185
violence
  Echinacea 161
visions

Lotus 72
vitality
    Calendula 154
    Rhododendron 106
vulnerable 178
    St-Johns-Wort 182
    Viburnum Burkwoodii 124
    White Rambling Rose 131
    Yellow-Poppy 140
warrior
    Mahonia 74
weakness
    Rhododendron 106
weary
    Blackthorn 149
    Sunshine Lift 237
weepiness
    Pulsatilla 178
wholeness

Pearl 193
will
    Pomegranate 102
wisdom
    Apple Blossom 26
    Clary-sage 159
    Willow 137
wise woman
    Black Cohosh 145
wonder
    Turkish-Filbert 123
workaholics
    Cornflower 41
worry
    Marsh-Mallow 173
    Scabious 114
youth
    Ox Eye Daisy 91

Printed in Great Britain
by Amazon